The Complete Book of
SLIMMING & DIETS

The Complete Book of
SLIMMING & DIETS

Dr Eric Trimmer

PIATKUS

© 1981 Dr Eric Trimmer

First published in 1981 by Judy Piatkus (Publishers) Limited
of Loughton, Essex

British Library Cataloguing in Publication Data

Trimmer, Eric
   The complete book of slimming and diets
   1. Reducing diets
   2. Physical fitness
   I. Title
   613.2'5   RM222.Z

ISBN 0-86188-081-1
ISBN 0-86188-116-8 paper

Designed by Mike Rose and Bob Lamb
Illustrations by Ken Stott and Mike Rose

Typeset by V & M Graphics Ltd., Aylesbury, Bucks.
Printed and bound by R. J. Acford Ltd., Chichester

Contents

Introduction

These days, you can almost guarantee that, if a group of about six friends gets together, at least one of them is on a diet, or has just been on a diet, or is just about to begin a diet. Practically every woman knows that depressing feeling when, not only is her normal dress-size too small, but the next one is a bit tight too. Many an executive becomes aware of just how many expense-account lunches he has consumed when he stands on the bathroom scales. Big is certainly *not* beautiful, nor, indeed, is it healthy. Overweight people are increasingly susceptible to a number of serious diseases and illnesses, some of which may even prove fatal. The grossly obese are at a very high risk and even the slightly overweight have measurably reduced their life expectancy.

It is hardly surprising, therefore, that diets and slimming are so widely discussed and so often written about. Advice and information bombards us from all sides and thousands of pounds have been poured into medical research into the problems, causes and cures of obesity. Yet, in spite of all this, the number of 'failed' dieters far exceeds the number of successful ones. *The Complete Book of Slimming and Diets* demonstrates that this need no longer be the case.

Right from the start, Dr Trimmer makes it clear that there is no-one, however fat, who *cannot* lose weight. He then goes on to explain how the body works, what foods are essential for good health and what creates extra, unnecessary and unwanted fat. He describes in detail how you can tell if you are overweight and by how much and helps to establish realistic target weights and timetables for achieving them.

The largest part of the book—and the most important—is devoted to the different kinds of diets. No single diet is right for everybody, but there is one that is absolutely right for you. Choosing a diet which matches your lifestyle and which you will enjoy following means that you will probably stick to it and succeed in losing that extra weight. Even more important, the right choice of diet will change your eating patterns so that you do not put the lost weight back on again immediately.

Each chapter looks at one single or

several related ways of losing weight and investigates the pros and cons. Clear and lucid explanations are backed up with graphs and charts. There are plenty of suggestions for diet meals to take the pain out of planning, including day-by-day menu guides and many easy-to-follow recipes.

In addition, a chapter is devoted to an investigation of the helpfulness and value of exercise as a means of losing weight. Dr Trimmer faces up to all the popular myths about exercise and brings the full weight of modern medical evidence to bear. You might be surprised to learn that you do not have to buy an expensive track suit and jog painfully around the park on winter mornings. You might be even more surprised to learn what a regular 30-minute walk can achieve. Helpful charts will show you at a glance the 'calorie-wasting' values of all kinds of exercise and sports.

Slimming groups have become very popular in the last ten years or so and Dr Trimmer looks at the ways they are organized and assesses the chances of success. He also gives a timely warning about other less honest and more expensive schemes designed to separate you from the pounds in your pocket rather than the pounds on your waistline.

Recognizing that even the most conscientious dieter is sometimes tempted to stray and that problems and difficulties may occur with any slimming regime, Dr Trimmer discusses the danger areas. He offers sensible advice and help if you are having problems and provides an invaluable list of diet-savers and substitute foods to help you over any sticky patches.

Finally, he answers a number of common questions about diets and slimming. On topics as varied as pregnancy, anorexia nervosa and slimming surgery, he draws on the most recent medical research taking place in Europe and America.

By the time you have finished reading *The Complete Book Slimming and Diets*, you will be able to make an informed decision about whether you need or want to lose weight, how much you should lose and how to go about it. The only thing this book cannot do for you is make the initial commitment to slim.

Diets at a glance

Other popular diets

Diets for healthy living

CHAPTER I

Anyone can slim

There is no-one, however fat, who cannot lose weight. Once you have decided to slim, choose the diet which will suit you best and stick to it. Diet adjustment is the key to successful slimming.

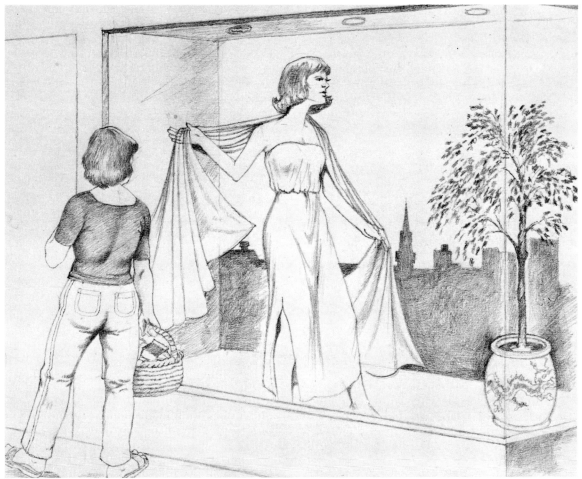

Fashions in figures and the perfect silhouette are constantly changing. The Marilyn Monroe figure is already passé and big is certainly not beautiful in our culture today. Awareness of obesity and a desire to be slim is not just a whim of the fashion designer and the media. To be overweight is unhealthy and it does not look attractive. It is also a bore and a nuisance when you outgrow your wardrobe, and can prove expensive when ready-to-wear clothes in the shops are sizes too small.

Putting on weight

People put on weight by eating food, more food than is needed. However, not every overweight person is a glutton, or even overeats very much. Often they eat no more than the person next door, their sister or their spouse (see Chapters III and XV). In cases like this, doctors talk of genetics and inborn traits. Some fat people have such an efficient digestive and food-absorbing facility

that they gain every little bit of nutriment from what they eat. It is a case of Nature working with the survival of the human race in mind. Suppose a nuclear bomb fell. The survivors of the devastation and subsequent famine would be the fatties—those so designed by Nature that they could scrape along and exist on a minimal intake of food.

Compulsive eating

Food is associated with feelings of comfort and security from infancy onwards. Some insecure people only show exactly how uncomfortable and insecure they are in their lives by the existence of their expanded waistlines. It is possible to go far enough along this line to reach a state where they have to keep eating to make life seem at all worthwhile. This gives the rest of us another label to hang around somebody else's neck and we call that person 'a compulsive eater'. These people do

11

not lose weight on their diet—all they lose is the diet sheet. They can only make a realistic decision to alter their eating patterns once their anxiety is under control. One such sufferer summed up the agony of the fat and nervous slimmer by remarking, 'If only I suffered from something that did not *show*.' The compulsive eater needs psychological help rather than a slimming regime, but the advice given in Chapter VII may prove helpful.

Compensation eating

There is also compensation eating. The classic case is that of the fictional Billy Bunter, who stuffed himself with chocolates and goodies because he hated school and his fellow pupils hated him. For Billy Bunter, 'tuck' was a compensation for his unhappiness. We discuss the problems of the fat child in Chapter X.

Some women are badly affected by the menopause and may overeat as a form of compensation for their lack of femininity (see Chapter XV).

Affluence can fatten

For some people, a fat stomach is like a Rolls Royce or a box at Ascot. This outward show of affluence can be a subconscious reason for being overweight—and liking it. Attitudes and life styles have changed. The affluent society has made us fat, almost as a side effect.

The way in which we spend our time has also changed. A lot of obesity is due to a couple of machines. The tiny but very efficient electric motor and the internal combustion engine. Think of your kitchen and your garden for a moment. Have you got a washing machine, a vacuum cleaner, an electric polisher, a food mixer, a power driven mower, an electric drill or a hedge clipper? If you have, fine. They take so much of the drudgery out of life. But every human benefit has to be paid for. Up goes your electricity bill and down goes the amount of energy you need to produce yourself. Up goes your body weight too, as saved energy expenditure is reflected in more food stored around your frame. What holds good for the kitchen and garden is increasingly true where general mobility is concerned. The advent, first of public transport and then of the car-a-person society has made tremendous changes in the way we use our body energy. Energy expenditure is discussed further in Chapter XII.

The effects of some of the changes and technical advances that have taken place in the last few decades are pretty subtle. Take central heating, for example. One way in which we use energy is to lose heat to our surroundings. Everyone, whether sitting in a train, working in an office, looking after home and family, even lying in bed, is like a small radiator. To keep your radiators at home hot, you pay for gas, oil or electricity. They lose heat to warm up the air around you. If you have a good central heating system, an efficient thermostat cuts off the source of energy when the room is hot enough and we, the walking radiators, do the same. The efficient thermostat is working away to keep down your energy bills and to keep up your bank balance. When the human radiator slows down, there is some evidence that the saved energy is added to the body's fat stores, Nature's bank balance for those possible difficult times ahead.

Are you too fat?

Some people do not know whether or not they should slim. Are they nicely covered or are they on the way to being overblown—inflated with excess fat? There are several ways to make sure which category you are in and the simplest is the pinch test. Doctors use calipers to measure this but fingers give a good enough guide and the result will tell you whether or not you should pursue the matter further. With your thumb and finger, take hold of the fleshy skin at the back of the top of your arm. If your finger and thumb are separated by more than 2 cm (¾ in) when you give yourself a good pinch, the chances are you are overweight. You should then do a more accurate check to find out exactly how overweight you are.

How overweight are you?

For many years, we (you, me, the dieticians and the doctors) have based our opinions of the 'right' weight on tables worked out by life insurance actuaries. Traditionally, these are divided into three varieties of body build, causing a dilemma in the dieter's mind—is he or she small, medium or large? It also leads to a curious state of affairs, whereby a variation of 18 kg (40 lb) is acceptable as the 'normal weight', of a tall man dependent upon his 'body build'. Such body build tables are now generally dismissed. A much more acceptable and accurate health test, based on height and weight, is derived from a simple formula resulting from very easy calculations. This is known as the Body Mass Index.

OLD-FASHIONED AND OUTMODED HEIGHT/WEIGHT TABLES

Desirable weight in pounds and *kilograms* (in indoor clothing), ages 25 and over

MEN

Height (in shoes)			Small frame		Medium frame		Large frame	
ft	in	*cm*	lb	*kg*	lb	*kg*	lb	*kg*
5	2	*157.5*	112-120	*50.8-54.4*	118-129	*53.5-58.5*	126-141	*57.2-64*
5	3	*160*	115-123	*52.2-55.8*	121-133	*54.9-60.3*	129-144	*58.5-65.3*
4	4	*162.6*	118-126	*53.5-57.2*	124-136	*56.2-61.7*	132-148	*59.9-67.1*
5	5	*165.1*	121-129	*54.9-58.5*	127-139	*57.6-63*	135-152	*61.2-68.9*
5	6	*167.6*	124-133	*56.2-60.3*	130-143	*59 -64.9*	138-156	*62.6-70.8*
5	7	*170.2*	128-137	*58.1-62.1*	134-147	*60.8-66.7*	142-161	*64.4-73*
5	8	*172.7*	132-141	*59.9-64*	138-152	*62.6.-68.9*	147-166	*66.7-75.3*
5	9	*175.3*	136-145	*61.7-65.8*	142-156	*64.4-70.8*	151-170	*68.5-77.1*
5	10	*177.8*	140-150	*63.5-68*	146-160	*66.2-72.6*	155-174	*70.3-78.9*
5	11	*180.3*	144-154	*65.3-69.9*	150-165	*68 -74.8*	159-179	*72.1-81.2*
6	0	*182.9*	148-158	*67.1-71.7*	154-170	*69.9-77.1*	164-184	*74.4-83.5*
6	1	*185.4*	152-162	*68.9-73.5*	158-175	*71.7-79.4*	168-189	*76.2-85.7*
6	2	*188*	156-167	*70.8-75.7*	162-180	*73.5-81.6*	173-194	*78.5-88*
6	3	*190.5*	160.171	*72.6-77.6*	167-185	*75.7-83.5*	178-199	*80.7-90.3*
6	4	*193*	164-175	*74.4-79.4*	172-190	*78.1-86.2*	182-204	*82.7-92.5*

WOMEN

Height (in shoes)			Small frame		Medium frame		Large frame	
ft	in	*cm*	lb	*kg*	lb	*kg*	lb	*kg*
4	10	*147.3*	92-98	*41.7-44.5*	96-107	*43.5-48.5*	104-119	*47.2-54*
4	11	*149.9*	94-101	*42.6-45.8*	98-110	*44.5-49.9*	106-122	*48.1-55.3*
5	0	*152.4*	96-104	*43.5-47.2*	101-113	*45.8-51.3*	109-125	*49.4-56.7*
5	1	*154.9*	99-107	*44.9-48.5*	104-116	*47.2-52.6*	112-128	*50.8-58.1*
5	2	*157.5*	102-110	*46.3-49.9*	107-119	*48.5-54*	115-131	*52.2-59.4*
5	3	*160*	105-113	*47.6-51.3*	110-122	*49.9-55.3*	118-134	*53.5-60.8*
5	4	*162.6*	108-116	*49 -52.6*	113-126	*51.3-57.2*	121-138	*54.9-62.6*
5	5	*165.1*	111-119	*50.3-54*	116-130	*49 -59*	125-142	*49.4-64.4*
5	6	*167.6*	114-123	*51.7-55.8*	120-135	*54.4-61.2*	129-146	*58.5-66.2*
5	7	*170.2*	118-127	*53.5-57.6*	124-139	*56.2-63*	133-150	*60.3-68*
5	8	*172.7*	122-131	*55.3-59.4*	128-143	*58.1-64.9*	137-154	*62.1-69.9*
5	9	*175.3*	126-135	*57.2-61.2*	132-147	*59.9-66.7*	141-158	*64 71.7*
5	10	*177.8*	130-140	*59 -63.5*	136-151	*61.7-68.5*	145-163	*65.8-73.9*
5	11	*180.3*	134-144	*60.8-65.3*	140-155	*63.5-70.3*	149-168	*67.6-76.2*
6	0	*182.9*	138-148	*62.6-67.1*	144-159	*65.3-72.1*	153-173	*69.4-78.5*

(From *Documenta Geigy Scientific Tables*, 7th edition, Basle, 1970)

This (metric) formula is body weight divided by height squared and can be written:

$$\frac{\text{Weight (in kg)}}{\text{Height}^2 \text{ (in cm)}}$$

Unless you are a mathematician, this is a difficult little sum to work out, but it takes about two seconds with a pocket calculator. For example, the calculations for a 94 kg man, 186 cm tall, will give the mysterious figure:

$$\frac{\text{Weight}}{\text{Height} \times \text{Height}} = \frac{94}{186 \times 186} = .00271708$$

The third and fourth figures on this scale are the relevant ones, in this case, 27.

A figure of 20 is taken as normal
25 to 30 is not too bad
30 to 40 is worrying
40+ is very dangerous

This new style gauge of normalcy is doubly interesting. First, it gives an indication of excess mortality due to overweight at all ages. Taking average mortality as being represented by 100, then

20 indicates 100 (average)
25 indicates an increased mortality of 142
35 indicates an increased mortality of 179

More details about the Body Mass Index in relation to mortality and illness are given in Chapter XV.

Second, it indicates approximately how long it will take to reach the ideal weight, with a low calorie diet of about 1,500 calories per day and if a reasonable exercise quotient is added to the diet.

25 to 30	3 to 6 months
30 to 40	6 to 10 months
40 plus	over 1 year

More details are given in Chapter XI.

The need to lose weight

We face a strange and quite modern dilemma. According to current research, between one quarter and one half of the population of most western-style societies feels the need to lose some weight. Predictably, this feeling of being too fat occurs just after Christmas and again when a summer holiday looms up on the not-too-distant horizon.

Unfortunately, there is no push-button way to slim, but, as we shall see, it is not too difficult to lose weight. To a large extent, the successful way to slim is to match the sort of person you are and the life you lead to the best method available that will suit you. Slimming means altering patterns of eating and activity. The different diets discussed in this book will help you to select the one that is right for you.

Why you should slim

The decision to slim is often reinforced by the knowledge that to be overweight is unhealthy, and just how unhealthy is discussed in Chapter XV. The list of illnesses associated with being overweight (backache, arthritis, varicose veins, digestive and metabolic disorders, diabetes, gallstones, cancer of the gall bladder, hernia, intestinal obstruction, stroke, thrombosis, coronary) reads like a medical horror story. But, like most other medical horror stories, such as 'smoking gives you lung cancer', the day when diabetes will strike or a coronary will lay you low is often many years ahead. Most health educators are belatedly discovering that medical horror stories in which the crunch comes a long way in the future rarely influence people and they do not change their unhealthy habits.

Some things do shake up the overweight and cause them to take action. For men, it is usually failing a medical examination for life insurance, or a sudden glance in the bathroom mirror. Women tend to slim for cosmetic or body image reasons.

Medical advice

There is the question of whether you should see a doctor before you start to diet or whether you should embark on a do-it-yourself regime. Slimming experts always like to be on the safe side and recommend that you should see a doctor if you are 6.5 kg (14 lb) overweight or if you know that you have something else wrong with you. That extra weight is not *always* caused by stores of fat being heaped on, gram by gram and ounce by ounce, over the years—only in about 99.9 per cent of cases!

The more potent slimming aids described in Chapter II are all prescription-only remedies and must be obtained through your doctor. Some doctors are very helpful about slimming and supply charts and diets on request, but a great many are not. They talk about 'will power' and 'what's on your body was on your plate' and they are not too concerned with ways of helping people to lose weight, although they all agree that to be overweight is unhealthy. There is no neat medical cure to the problem of obesity and this makes doctors today behave rather unhelpfully. So, for most slimmers, it is a question of do it yourself or do nothing. However, if you are seriously overweight, do not go on a crash diet or three-day fast without first consulting a doctor.

Are extra vitamins necessary?

Most doctors advise slimmers to take a good multivitamin pill each day. There is a certain amount of evidence that thiamin (a B complex vitamin) helps in converting food to energy rather than storing it as fat. No good slimmer should be without it. High fat dieters can be a little short of vitamin C and, although we do not actually see scurvy breaking out in the ranks of slimmers, a daily dose of Vitamin C can do no harm and may well be beneficial.

Some low calorie diets are also very low in fat and, therefore, low in the essential fat soluble vitamins A and D. Cod-liver oil is Nature's best source of these vitamins. It also contains supplies of substances called essential fatty acids, which the body cannot make out of ordinary animal fat but which, nevertheless, are very necessary for good health. The remedy is obvious. You should take two cod-liver oil capsules a day if you are on one of the low fat diets in addition to the multi-vitamin pill.

Some slimmers find that their hair becomes lifeless or dull when they are on a diet and this can make them feel lifeless and dull too. This means that the slimming programme is pretty well on the rocks of failure. Cod-liver oil's essential fatty acids get into the hair follicles and improve the way the hair looks. There are definitely some diets that need extra vitamins to give the best results in terms of feeling fit and looking good.

How difficult is it to lose weight?

It can be easy or difficult to lose weight, depending on your approach. Some overweight people approach their slimming with a sense of grim foreboding—and no wonder. Eating is one of life's great pleasures for most of us. If we did not enjoy it and feel bad when we were hungry, the human race would have died out years ago. But it is quite possible, and fairly easy, to *adjust* your eating pattern so that, instead of getting fatter every day, you get slimmer without the pangs of hunger. The key word is adjustment.

It would be a good idea if we could lose the word *diet* from our language. The very words, 'I'm on a diet,' or 'I've got to go on a diet,' sound like bad news and most people regard going on a diet with the same enthusiasm as they do a trip to the dentist or the bank manager. Actually the word diet crept into our language from the French in the middle of the sixteenth century and means *to regulate oneself as to eating*. So it seems that we are stuck with it. Before this, to diet simply meant to feed and it is this feeding aspect of slimming on which this book concentrates.

Painful and punitive 'dieting' must go out of the window because it just does not work with normal people. Slimming here means losing weight by adjusting your food intake. It is a game everyone can play—and enjoy winning.

Before you reach for your first piece of crispbread, here are two mottos to hang up on the wall of your subconscious mind.
1 **One good diet that you can stick to is worth ten half-hearted diets that you only play at for a few weeks.**
2 **The bigger your problem (in terms of weight to be lost) the longer it will take to solve—but this does not mean that it will be more difficult to solve.**

According to research, it is easier to lose weight if you are a young man, a first-time dieter, have a stable personality, have an interesting social life and are reasonably affluent. But for every person who finds himself so happily placed, there are hundreds who do not. They, too, can slim successfully.

Mental attitude

Often, lack of will-power is given as a reason for not slimming or for failing at slimming. The phrase, 'I've no will-power,' somehow absolves the slimmer from bad feelings about weight-loss.

Perhaps it evokes the vision of a rather racy and attractive inability to resist temptation in all sorts of other ways too. In fact, 'will-power' is not necessary to successful slimming. All that is necessary is to make a decision. Once you have made up your mind, then voicing your decision to lose weight to family, friends, at the office or slimming club is a useful aid to weight reduction. Making a public announcement to encourage yourself to maintain a plan of action is an ancient and helpful tradition. If you go back on your word, everybody is likely to take things you say in the future less seriously. As the orientals say you lose face.

Remember, you and you alone have control over your own stomach. Some people find that to diet with a friend, colleague or spouse makes them more determined to succeed. It can add an element of healthy competition and makes it more difficult to cheat. Others find that a wager with friends gives an extra incentive. Many more choose to join a slimming group (see Chapter VII).

Sometimes, people who talk about having no will-power for slimming are actually talking in code. What they are really saying is, 'There's an advantage to me in being fat, but I'm not telling *you* about it! Or even *me*!'

The golden rules of weight reduction

The motivation factor   This is possibly the most important thing to learn about slimming. There must be a meaningful, personal reason for the slimmer to lose weight. Doctors may advise and friends may urge but, for the slimmer to move into the weight-loss success group, the decision has to be entirely personal. Whatever the reason, the decision to lose weight must be 100 per cent enthusiastic and personal.

If you really want to lose weight you can and it is relatively easy. If you are half-hearted about it from the start, then have a nice fattening jam sandwich and forget all about it.

The time factor   Even the most stable and self-confident person experiences times in his life when self-discipline and a change in behaviour will be difficult. This is not the time to start on weight reduction. Solve problems and assuage anxieties first; then slim.

The reduction factor   Set a goal and make it a realistic one. Base your target weight on average

weight tables, if you like. Alternatively, aim for the weight you were before you had to abandon all those clothes that used to fit you so nicely. Realistic slimming goals rather than vague fantasy breed success.

You cannot beat the clock   You get fat at a steady rate for you and you will slim at about the same rate. Certain crash diets, gimmicky diets and exotic cures will often make you seem to be shedding pounds at an amazing rate. The chances are that you will be losing weight in the form of body fluids, not fat. The body will compensate for this fluid loss by retaining more fluid and in three weeks' time you will be back where you started.

Earlier the better   The sooner you slim the more likely you are to succeed. The task does not seem so enormous and the goal is reached quicker.

Choose the right diet for you   To be effective, a diet has to meet all the slimmer's nutrient needs *except* the fattening factors. Not matching the diet to the person is perhaps the commonest reason for slimming failure. Almost all successful diets contain the following points.
1 **They take into account the tastes and habits of the potential slimmer.**
2 **They protect against hunger between meals.**
3 **They provide a sense of well-being without fatigue.**
4 **They are acceptable 'at home and away' but do not encourage a feeling of being 'different' or 'odd'.**
5 **They are designed to encourage a new way of eating so that, once the goal is reached and more food is permissible, a lifetime of eating without gaining weight is maintained.**

Is there a best diet for you?

Of course there is a diet suited to your special needs. In fact, more slimmers fail because they have embarked on the wrong sort of diet than for any other reason. In the following chapters, you will find many diet options and the information that will help you select the easiest and most effective slimming diet for you.

You need to lose your stored body fat in order to lose weight. The object of each diet is to make the body use its stored fat to produce energy. This is achieved by means of food intake adjustment and helped by increased energy expenditure.

The three most popular ways to adjust your

eating pattern and effect weight-loss are the low carbohydrate, high fat and high protein diets.

The low carbohydrate diets given in Chapters III and IV are excellent in terms of general nutrition and well-being. The individual diets described are not all strictly calorie controlled but there is an emphasis on healthy eating.

The high fat diet described in Chapter V can be a real gourmet's delight. It virtually eliminates carbohydrates from the diet and concentrates on a high fat intake, with plenty of butter, cream and fatty meats. This speeds up the metabolism and results in a quick weight-loss. People who choose to follow this dietary regime usually find it easy to keep to because there is no cause to feel hungry.

The high protein diet is discussed in Chapter VI, and modifications are referred to throughout the book. It is particularly suitable for children, adolescents and those who enjoy fairly regular business lunches. It is a fact that the more protein you eat, the more you 'waste'. A high protein diet gives a rapid initial weight-loss, which is a very satisfactory way to start a diet. A dieter following this regime will never feel hungry. However, high protein foods do tend to be expensive.

Information is given on other forms of dieting, including low fat and 'free' diets, high-fibre carbohydrate diets, diets suitable for slimming groups and for healthy living. They will all introduce you to a new pattern of eating which you can follow, and enjoy, for life.

Many slimming books baldly state 'Do it my way!' Sometimes their ways help but, if they do not, it is because those ways are wrong for you. How, for instance, can a high fat diet help you if you cannot stand fat at any price? Counting calories will be hopeless if counting anything makes your head spin. Quite often finances come into dieting and there are cheap diets and relatively expensive ones. An example of a low expenditure diet is the meat extract diet given in Chapter III. By contrast, paying a lot to slim can sometimes help. Plain simple eaters will not feel at ease for very long on a gourmet diet. The rather introspective aspects to some diets are not suitable for the extrovert who does not really care for observing the body quite so carefully.

To start with, while you are learning about diets and slimming, keep an open mind. Learn a little about how your body works before you make the adjustments necessary to reduce body weight. We are all very different in numerous ways. Our personal preferences are part of us. Indulge them while slimming. It pays handsome dividends.

Why so many different diets?

Slimming books and magazines have now become a growth industry and the reason for this is quite obvious. A constant supply of new ideas is needed because so many slimmers fail with one technique and want to try another. Only about one-quarter of those who go on a slimming diet enjoy success and even that meagre 25 per cent do not maintain their weight reduction for very long.

Most obese people who undertake weight reduction will not keep on with the diet. Of those who do, most will not lose much weight. Of those who do lose weight, most will regain it quite soon. This is one realistic summary of the slimming business.

A global review of slimming 'cures' reached the following depressing conclusion. Only one in four people who start slimming end up by losing 9 kg (20 lb) and only five per cent lose as much as 18 kg (40 lb). However, this discouraging state of affairs can be looked at another way. The 25 per cent of slimmers who succeeded in losing 9 kg (20 lb) are roughly the same sort of animal as the rest of us. Their success must point the way out of the depressing 75 per cent failure figure. Studying the successful slimmers and their diets tells us all we want to know about slimming.

Body types and suitable diets

We all start life as a single cell, which divides into two and then into four and so on. Before he is even a few days old, a developing baby looks a bit like a blackberry under the microscope. But already the individual cells are starting to differentiate or specialize. On the outside of the 'blackberry' are cells that will become the skin, brain and nervous system. These cells are called ectoderm or outside skin. In the centre of this little ball of cells is an inner layer, the endoderm, which will become the digestive system and bowels. In between is the mesoderm, which eventually develops into bone and muscle.

What has all this to do with slimming? Well, not very much, but it is slightly relevant and surprisingly important. As we develop into people, sometimes we seem to be dominated by one or another sort of tissue. This has led doctors to classify certain people as predominantly having particular body types. The ectomorphic person is slightly built and has a finely tuned and dominant nervous system. Ectomorphs are quick, jumpy and clever—successful business people or sometimes sportsmen, jockeys and golfers. They seldom have weight problems and are, generally, not much interested in food and drink. The predominantly ectomorphic men and women are the keep-thins who do not need this book very much anyway.

The opposite body type is endomorphic. Endomorphs' digestive systems function well and easily. They like and are interested in food. They have large lips and efficient mouths. They tend to move slowly, are friendly, loving and chubby by nature. The pure endomorph will gain weight easily and will often need to exercise dietary control all through his or her lifetime.

The mesomorph is Mr Muscle Man on the beach or the sporty girl who loves physical activity. Mesomorphs are usually on the heavy side but their weight is healthy, for it is mostly muscle. Their eating patterns are usually those of good trenchermen, without gourmet tastes or a passion for beautifully cooked, elegant food. They eat to keep fit and well so that they can flex their muscles and enjoy plenty of athletic movement. Usually they maintain a constant weight until middle age when, because they do not take so much exercise, their healthy, indiscriminate appetite tends to encourage obesity, unless they reduce their total food intake to their new levels of activity.

The majority of people fall somewhere in between these body types. The modern fashion in dietetics is to soft pedal these body types, or somatotypes, as they are called. My opinion is that you can never know too much about yourself, if you or your family are overweight and need a diet, and all relevant knowledge has a useful application in this fascinating, if rather difficult, subject.

As mentioned above, ectomorphs do not need diet books. Often their families wish that they could gain some weight, feeling mistakenly that the ectomorph's inherent slimness indicates frailty or a tendency towards certain diseases. Nothing could be further from the truth. Usually ectomorphs are tough and fit, despite their lean and hungry appearance.

Endomorphs, in their constant weight battle, need very well thought-out diets that concentrate on giving gastronomic treats. A cleverly worked out and elaborate calorie counting diet often suits them and they will cheerfully spend hours comparing avocado pears, oysters and smoked salmon on this score. Often they do very well on high fat, low carbohydrate diets.

Mesomorphs always want to look after their muscles. They do not thrive on calorie counting diets as a slimming aid. Sometimes these deplete body protein, especially if a football playing mesomorph has recently joined the touchline and put on about 19 kg (42 lb) as a result. High protein, low carbohydrate diets are the answer for overweight mesomorphs.

Does age and sex matter?

Age and sex seem to be mentioned in relation to almost everything these days. To what extent do they influence slimming or being overweight? In the same way that children experience growth spurts during their development, so there are plumpness spurts at all ages. They can iron themselves out naturally. In adolescent girls, puppy fat usually falls off with the onset of regular menstruation. However, there is a tendency for all of us to put on weight at about forty and 'middle-aged spread', unchecked, can remain with us until the age of about 65, when Nature slims us down again. Some elderly people get quite thin without changing their eating habits very much. Sex comes into slimming, too. Men can lose weight much more easily than women.

To some extent, age and sex can dictate the diet you choose. Children and adolescents should use the high protein method of losing weight. They need all the muscle-building bricks of nutrition they can get, but only a handful or so of carbohydrate calories. People over sixty should not try a high fat diet because they may experience difficulty in digesting fat in large quantities.

Can dieting make you look worse?

'I'd love to slim but it makes me look terrible. My neck gets scraggy, my stomach sags and my bottom looks as big as ever.' This woman's predicament is fairly common and in such situations doctors are tempted to trot out that lovely piece of medical jargon, 'It's a pity you didn't come to see me sooner.' However, it is necessary to explain to the dieter that everybody stores fat rather individually, in special places. There are many curious machines sold today which claim to help with 'spot slimming', but unfortunately they do not create beautiful figures (see Chapter XIII).

Slow dieting, as opposed to going for quick weight-loss, minimizes that haggard look which can easily kill slimming enthusiasm. Diets which induce ketosis (discussed below) accentuate the haggard look. If you find that you lose too much weight around the neck and face, do not persevere with a ketosis-inducing diet but go for a more balanced diet, such as the week of slimming meals suggested in Chapter III.

Exercise combined with a diet will help you to look better. Exercise rebuilds the body, muscle-wise, as the fat drops off. We discuss the benefits of exercise in a slimming programme later in the book.

Finally, it is a good idea for those people who make a considerable investment in slimming to make an equal investment at the clothes shop. Your new body needs some nice new things to make it look good in its new shape. This applies to men as well as to women. And if you find that your hair becomes dull and lifeless when you are on a diet, that is a problem easily solved. Take a couple of cod-liver oil capsules each day.

Does dieting make you feel bad?

Some dieting can make you feel horrid, but slimming by diet adjustment does not. Hunger is an unpleasant sensation. There is an unease associated with it that is difficult to describe. It makes babies cry and can be experienced as a pain or a pang by us all. There is an element of body chemistry associated with hunger in that we experience the sensation when our blood sugar is low. There is also a slightly mysterious element of habit and timing about it. Anybody who has had his internal time clock upset by a long jet flight, when days and nights are jumbled together, tends to find himself waking up in the middle of the night ready for a three course meal, or sitting down to lunch with no appetite at all.

Crash diets or fast introductions to dieting (see Chapter IV) can make you feel pretty terrible if you opt for them in the wrong circumstances. Never try to soldier on and work normally if you are on a dietary nose-dive into only a few hundred calories a day.

One good tip for people who feel ill when they are on a diet, particularly at the beginning, is to eat twice as many *small* meals a day as they do at the moment. Provided that no more food is eaten, the greater the number of eating periods per day the better the weight-loss. Eating actually uses up energy as well as stoking up the fires of metabolism to help you slim.

There are various ways in which the pangs of hunger can be assuaged. Usually they can be tricked to go away and all good slimming routines have anti-hunger tricks built into them. Often something that tastes sweet, like a slim-line or diet drink will do it. Alternatively, something that makes the stomach feel 'full', like a glass of water, a cup of soup or some bran can help (see Chapter XI). Other anti-hunger tricks, or slimming aids, are discussed in the next chapter. They can also help to speed up the slimming process.

Ketosis

One anti-hunger device, built into many good slimming schemes is a phenomenon called ketosis. We lose weight by losing stored body fat. To slim we make our body use fat for producing energy, by means of food adjustments. On very low carbohydrate diets, fat does not entirely burn up into energy and water in the same way as carbohydrate does. Some partially burnt up fat (ketones) starts to accumulate in the blood. When this reaches a certain level, it is excreted from the body in the urine and, to some extent, in the breath too. One woman while she was slimming used to get her husband to smell her breath! When it smelt 'ketone sweet', he could reassure her that her diet was working.

The interesting thing is that ketosis often takes away the appetite and is a great aid to slimming. Some people find that ketosis makes them feel a bit odd for a few days. Nervous and anxious slimmers may interpret this as an indication that their new eating pattern is making them ill. Consequently, they go back to their previous way of life and become, of course, failed slimmers. This is a pity, for ketosis never harmed anybody who was otherwise fit and well. Not all slimmers experience ketosis as a nasty sensation. For some the feeling is new and rather attractive. One slimmer called it her 'slimming high', a part of slimming she really enjoyed. For most of us, ketosis is a 'different' feeling, neither unpleasant nor a wild slimming 'fix', but something in between. Some very effective diets measure ketosis by means of urine tests to monitor dieting (see Chapter VIII).

Hunger, that uneasy feeling that can reduce a baby from a peaceful and beautiful being into a wild squawking bundle of humanity in about fours hour flat, has another strange characteristic. After about 24 hours starvation, it changes radically, perhaps mainly due to ketosis. This is why hunger strikers do not feel the pain that might be expected.

Reasons for remaining overweight

When people ask doctors how they should slim, doctors may reply, 'Why do you want to stay fat?' One man quoted his wife. 'It's a good thing you are fat,' she had said. 'At your height you would look quite ridiculous if you were skinny.' He really had a weight problem. Some people reason that they must be basically fit if they are fat. They often have worries about wasting diseases, such as cancer and tuberculosis, lurking in the backs of their minds. These worries must be explored in some detail in order to make them realise the importance of losing weight.

There are many subconscious reasons for feeling good about being overweight.

Being a good boy and pleasing mother It does not matter how logical or bright you are, the fact remains that you were programmed in your childhood and the things that your mother taught you are buried deeply in your psyche. 'If you don't eat you'll get ill,' and 'If you don't eat your dinner you won't be big and strong like daddy, or a nice and loving person like mummy,' are messages and implications frequently repeated to children, even by the 'best' parents. They tend to be absorbed and stored away for future reference in the world's most receptive computer—a child's brain. Perhaps years later, the subconscious mind feeds in a request for information on a worrying subject to the computer-like brain. For example, 'What makes me ill, feel weak or even incapable of being loving?' Out come the answers: 'Illness strikes if you don't eat well. Loving comforting people eat well. If you don't eat you get weak.' To avoid being influenced by these feelings you have to recognize that they exist.

I'm big even if I'm not strong Some fat people subconsciously see their fat and their shapeless flabby bodies—something that they may profess to hate—as a semblance of strength and power. Weight reduction makes them feel weak and insignificant so, naturally, they do not slim.

I'm fat and therefore sexually safe A fear of being attractive sexually is not all that uncommon and obesity then becomes a useful 'turn-off' and protection against prospective suitors. Remaining fat and unattractive and giving a good excuse for it, such as lack of will-power, means a release from the problem of forming emotional attachments and behaving sexually.

I'm getting even with you Getting a 'kick' out of being overweight is not unusual. It is common in children and teenagers, but this ingeniously coded behaviour crops up in adulthood too. By being a 'disgrace to look at', the fat person 'strikes back' at others in a curious way. Unable to express hostility in more usual ways, the 'pain' that he or she inflicts on others by being 'disgustingly fat' is a useful way of obtaining retaliation for real or supposed injustices.

I'm a disgusting person anyway In some psychological states, self-punishment is necessary for emotional survival. The masochistic self justification is that overweight and looking terrible is a punishment for being a dreadful person. Coupled with this obesity is a cry for help: 'Can't you see I need sympathy, help and protection?' In such cases, 'How can I succeed, be liked, or do good with this terrible body?' is encoded into 'I can't lose weight, I haven't got the will-power.' For slimmers to hope to succeed while having made these 'package deals' with themselves is totally unrealistic.

Body image

It is worth understanding about body image factors because they give us insight into many of the mysteries of slimming failure and success. How we see ourselves is often unrelated to how we look to others. This can be a major influence on slimming.

Negative aspects

Some people review weight reduction as a threat to their total body integrity and image of self. A slimmer who says disapprovingly, 'I hardly recognized myself in the mirror, I look so different' (after dieting) is commenting on his body image. Some dieters, if asked to alter a photograph of themselves (as they really are) to make it look more like them, by means of a distorting lens, always adjust it to look fatter. Such people have difficulty in sticking to a slimming routine because they always tend to overestimate their body size and so reinforce their comforting 'self' concepts. This is called the 'phantom body size phenomenon'. Such people, when slimming, perceive themselves as having almost no weight, despite what the scales say. Naturally they tend to give up their diets.

Others with body image problems see their

bodies as just another object in the world around them, like a chair or a table—something apart from their real inner selves. For years, they may have viewed this 'object body' with amusement or even tenderness. If, however, as a result of something they read or are told about, they suddenly glimpse their bodies as the real central core of themselves, they are overwhelmed with anxiety, self contempt or even self hatred. This confrontation of image with true body self is so terrifying that they are forced towards one of two ways to deal with the nasty feeling. They may assume a role of physical illness. Sometimes the psychic package deal is, 'I'm fat because I'm ill.' Commonly, this illness role remains as a comforting defence against any further change of body image or slimming. Alternatively they take a positive approach, as in the case of the fat photographer described below.

It is not a good idea to try to pressurize people with body image problems into dieting and weight reduction. The anxiety and depression liable to follow has as much, if not more, to do with developing heart disease, blood pressure and so on as being overweight has. An emotional stability assessment should be a prerequisite of any slimming diet for middle-aged women, who most frequently pose such body image symptoms.

Recent work has shown that trying to persuade such women to slim can be disastrous, particularly to their sexual lives and happiness. In such a woman, plumpness allows her to relax and enjoy sex because she is not starving for food. These plump, comfortable women are used to experimenting and enjoying gourmet pleasures in the field of human sexuality as well as at the table. It has been said, perhaps rather unkindly, that the plump woman learns how to be more seductive so that she can compete with her conventionally more attractive, slim-line sisters. This may or may not be the case. Nevertheless, there seems little doubt that a fat person, male or female, who has succeeded in losing weight without solving body image problems has more emotional and sexual difficulty than other people.

Positive aspects

The sudden self-consciousness that erupts when someone is confronted with his body image as a real part of himself is not always followed by anxiety, depression or a retreat into illness, but by another natural reaction. A well publicized example is the story of the fat photographer, Bob Adelman.

Bob Adelman, who weighed 138 kg (305 lb), decided to photograph himself to see how he looked to others. The sudden confrontation of his photographic body image and his body image concept shocked him profoundly. He enrolled at a slimming clinic which specialized in group therapy and a diet/exercise slimming regime with some novel features. He took a series of photographs of himself over the following nine months and his changed body image reinforced his slimming goals. At the end of his slimming period he weighed 86 kg (190 lb) and his body image was excellent.

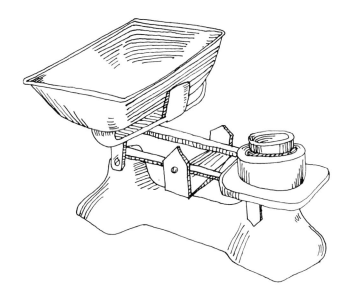

CHAPTER II

Slimming aids

Slimming aids can help to speed up the slimming process. Drugs and bulk fillers reduce the appetite and many people find the wide range of proprietary slimming foods very useful.

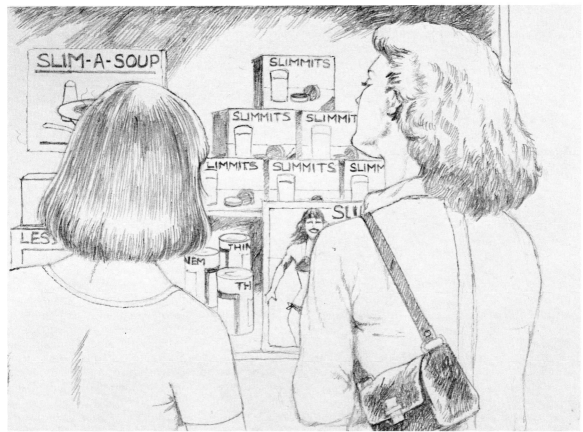

The best slimming 'aid' is probably medical advice. This medical advice can come from several sources—an interested doctor, a dietician, a psychologist who understands slimming, even a philosopher or a good book on the subject.

Generally, doctors disapprove of slimming aids, which is rather a pity. Dieters and slimming clinics, on the other hand, quite often find them helpful. You can slim without them, but some people find that they speed up the process.

Most slimming aids have one major snag. The body is an ingenious chemical factory and does not like having to deal with strange, unnatural chemicals floating about in the circulation. Consequently, it produces detoxifying substances (enzymes) which break down such compounds into simple, harmless substances. It can then get rid of them in the usual ways—mostly by excreting them in the urine.

Most slimming pills work because they are drugs which cause loss of appetite as a side effect. To start with, this loss of appetite is very noticeable because the body is slow to manufacture the detoxifying agents. Gradually the

body learns the knack of detoxifying slimming aids rapidly. Therefore, after about three weeks, or longer with some types, they no longer affect the appetite so much. A few slimming aids have addictive or potentially addictive qualities. They alter how we *feel* as well as how hungry we are. The feeling they promote is a pleasurable one. Some slimmers become addicted to such pills quite quickly and feel very bad indeed if their supply is cut off.

Bulk fillers

Celevac, Cellucon and Nilstim are cellulose tablets which absorb water after being swallowed. They swell up and expand in the stomach and are said, therefore, to reduce appetite. Critics claim that they swell so slowly they do not reach their full bulk until after they have left the stomach. One well respected researcher, however, found that relatively large doses, given as part of a diet programme, produced a better weight-loss than the diet did alone.

A snag is that they can have a laxative effect.

There is no risk of addiction and the safety factor is high.

Prefil contains sterculia and guangum. It is similar to cellulose fillers, but made in granule form for easier swallowing.

Bulk fillers are available from a chemist.

Proprietary foods

There are a great number of proprietary foods offered as slimming aids. Some of these offer fairly expensive and rather dull food as an alternative to the more ordinary things that we eat. Others substitute meals with special drinks and biscuits, which have the same calorific value as ordinary food. For those who feel that a financial investment is the price they must 'pay' in order to keep to a slimming regime, then proprietary slimming foods can be of use. But all too often they are a four-week wonder—a disappointing weight-loss over four weeks which is regained in (you've guessed it) the next four weeks as your body compensates.

Recommended are the excellent range of slimming soups which are now available, low-calorie drinks and also the 'something to munch at', no-calorie slimming aids available on the chemist's shelves. Low-calorie bars of chocolate are well worth trying if you enjoy sweet things. They can also act as an appetite suppressor. 'Low-calorie' breads and crispbreads are, in fact, high in calories. However, they are light and are of benefit if taken in fairly small quantities. For those who find their will of iron changing at the drop of a hat (or the smell of a hamburger) to the consistency of eggshell, these aids to slimming do have a part to play. Browsing around in your local chemist's shop and sorting them out can also take the edge off your appetite.

Artificial sweeteners

Artificial sweeteners are frowned upon in several parts of the world at the moment. Almost every tried and tested sugar substitute has its own particular horror story concerning what happened to some poor unfortunate group of rats in a laboratory where they ate the sweeteners by the ton for months on end. Many doctors have a built-in resistance to investigative journalism, based on a working knowledge of those who do the investigating and a great deal of information on the vested interests of all those involved.

Ideally, for people with a sweet tooth, a gradual re-education directed towards exploring the ways of altering flavour preference in favour of savoury rather than sweet foods is indicated. But if you find coffee and tea without sugar too unpalatable, then use any of the proprietary sweeteners and forget about the white mouse medicine horror stories.

Amphetamine and related drugs

Experiments have shown that slimmers on constant calorie diets lose more weight if they are given amphetamines. It seems that this weight-loss is due to increased restlessness and a speeding up of activity. People on free eating schedules plus amphetamines lose weight mostly due to loss of appetite. A feeling of well-being, called euphoria, complicates the picture, however, as this pleasant sensation is only maintained by relentlessly increasing the dose of the drug. To obviate this, chemists played 'molecular roulette' with the amphetamine molecule in an attempt to find an amphetamine-like drug with no addictive properties. With the exception of a few compounds, they have not succeeded.

The safety factor is low and amphetamines can be addictive in some people. They are available on prescription only.

'Safe' amphetamines

Scientific statistics show that usually, but not always, slimmers on free diets lose weight when taking the 'safe' amphetamines, Apisate and Tenuate. Some side effects have to be accepted. Restlessness, dry mouth and constipation are common. Feelings of euphoric well-being are rare, but dependence has occasionally been reported. (Drug dependence is a complicated subject. Some addicts become 'dependent' on almost any drug, even those with extremely unpleasant side effects.) These two drugs work quite well in on-off routines which mitigate against habituation. For the very obese, they are helpful and are effective for a long while (about 24 weeks) before the body learns to detoxify them.

The safety factor is fairly good. Also, these drugs can be used by slimmers suffering from hypertension and heart disease. 'Safe' amphetamines may be prescribed by your doctor.

Ionamin is a quick and effective slimming aid but it is of moderate duration. Unfortunately, undesirable side effects can occur. Amphetamine-like 'highs' are relatively common and hallucinations have been reported.

The safety factor is only poor to fair. Ionamin is unsuitable for slimmers undergoing anti-hypertension or certain anti-depression treatments.

Ponderax is unique in that, although it is closely related to amphetamine chemically, there are no stimulating side effects. In fact, it has a curiously sedative action. Ponderax is excellent for the very obese and a full nine months' usage is necessary before the drug becomes ineffective as a slimming aid. The worst thing about Ponderax is its plethora of side effects. These include tummy pains and diarrhoea, dizziness and dry mouth. Rarely, slimmers may feel depressed when they stop taking Ponderax. It acts to help weight-loss in various ways. It reduces appetite and it tends to 'mobilize' body fat and partially to block the manufacture of fats from carbohydrates. Ponderax is especially useful when obesity is associated with anxiety. It can help the anxious eater, provided he can tolerate the side effects.

The safety factor is high. Ponderax can be used by slimmers with high blood pressure, except when they are taking certain anti-hypertensive drugs. Special medical precautions are necessary in cases of depression, diabetes and pregnancy.

A non-amphetamine aid

Teronac is a compound unrelated chemically to amphetamines, but which has a selective, amphetamine-like action. Its appetite suppressing action is similar to amphetamine. It can also cause euphoria, but only if it is improperly used and taken in large quantities. It remains effective for 16 weeks as a slimming aid, but it is not free from side effects, which include agitation and sometimes insomnia. It often causes a rise in blood pressure and pulse rate.

The safety factor is good, but Teronac is unsuitable for slimmers with peptic ulcer, glaucoma, coronary disease or anxiety. It is also unsuitable for slimmers taking antihypertensive drugs or those undergoing certain depression treatments. Teronac is available on a doctor's prescription only.

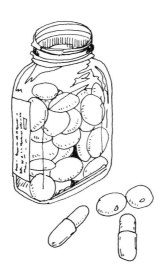

CHAPTER III

What makes you fat?

Doctors and dieticians recognize that there are two types of people—those who put on weight very easily and those who don't. To understand diets and slimming and to know what makes people fat, it is necessary to have a basic knowledge of nutrition and the carbohydrate and calorie content of foods.

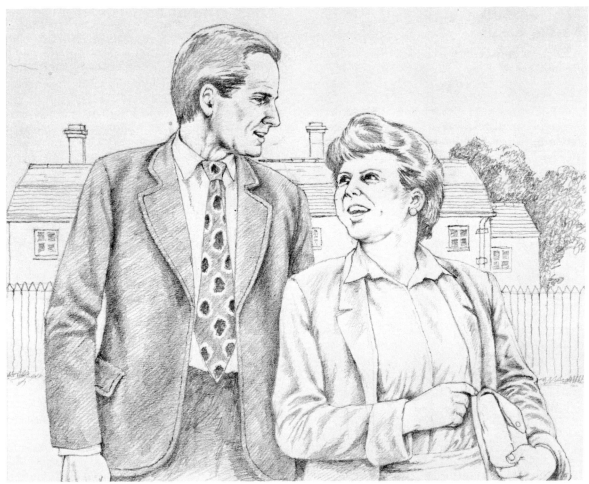

'Why is it that my husband eats and drinks much more than I do and never puts on any weight, and yet, if I indulge myself a little, in a few weeks I cannot get into any of my clothes?' Numerous variations of this plaintive question are asked by overweight people all the time, the world over. All too often, the doctor or the dietician compounds the agony by saying something to the effect that every kilogram on your body comes off the plate or out of a glass. It is, of course, true but it does nothing to answer the question or to help the slimmer.

The true answer to the question is 'there is no one answer'. In fact, the doctors and dieticians, if they are really honest, now say, 'Some of the answers we previously gave were fairly wild guesses. We believed them to be true in the past, but now we know better.' Of course, there are some types of obesity that are very well understood. For example there is an obesity 'centre' in the brain, called the hypothalamus, and tumours, injury and inflammation, with meningitis, for instance, affecting this area, cause quite startling 'hypothalamic' obesity. There are also a few glandular types of obesity. Alterations of the function of the adrenal glands (over the kidney) and the pancreas (under the stomach) are sometimes followed by relentless obesity. Changes in sex-gland function can tip some people into obesity quite quickly—for instance, castration, the change of life or even pregnancy. More detailed information is given in Chapter XV. A few rare cases of obesity are genetic. Certain drugs, such as oestrogens, used in the contraceptive pill and for hormone replacement therapy, and phenothiazines, used in psychiatry, are associated with weight gain in some people.

However, these causes of obesity are not common and the main causes are probably inactivity and food intake in people whose bodies contain something which is not clearly understood but may be called a 'fatten easily' factor.

Mr Constant Weight and Mrs Fatten Easily

A fairly simplistic way to look at the problem is to assume there are two types of people - the husband and the wife who posed the leading question. The husband—Mr Constant Weight—can adjust his internal metabolic fires to match his food intake. Even if he eats masses of fattening, carbohydrate food his weight stays steady, because his body merely increases its internal burning up of food process (metabolic rate). Mrs Fatten Easily only stays at a constant weight if she matches her food intake accurately to her energy expenditure. Extra food is quickly converted into fat and stored on her body.

This is a neat, little theory and, like many such convenient explanations, it suffers from one disadvantage. There is very little scientific evidence in human beings that proves or disproves it. Many rather haphazard studies, which were neither very well designed nor controlled, have been carried out. They were mostly variations on a single, basic theme. A nutrition scientist gives a vast supply of chocolate to a group of people, usually medical students, who often act as 'guinea pigs' in this type of study. They are instructed to eat a fixed weight of chocolate each day in addition to their normal food intake. They are weighed before the study starts and again after several weeks. Some are found to have gained weight and some have not. At a quick glance, it seems that the theory that some people fatten easily has been proved. A more sceptical look, however, shows that the experiment is not really telling us very much. For instance, did all the students really add the extra calorie-packed chocolate to their everyday diet? Did some, perhaps, unconsciously and due to lack of appetite, eat less of their ordinary food while they were chocolate gorgers? The experiment also tells us little about the students' activities—both their total (exercise) activity and the speed at which they went about things. Activity does strange things to fat storage. Generally, increased food intake plus reduced activity equals weight increase. However, from studies of some birds, we know that decreased food intake in the late summer and autumn plus normal activity will produce a 50 per cent weight gain. When we really understand facts like this, we will know considerably more about obesity and more about the differences between Mr Constant Weight and Mrs Fatten Easily.

The Vermont Experiment

There is at least one human experiment that does give some support, as well as some criticism of the Mr Constant Weight and Mrs Fatten Easily theory. A group of young and normally lean prisoners at the Vermont State Prison, U.S.A., volunteered to embark upon a controlled 'fattening up' experiment. A special dining room, kitchen facilities, recreation and television room were installed. The prison hospital medical organization and warders supervised the whole system, in conjunction with the Professor of Medicine at Vermont University. The volunteers were encouraged to overeat and the amount of food, the composition of the diet and their activity were carefully logged and controlled. The results of this survey were extremely interesting, for it showed that most, but not all, of the volunteers gained weight by increased food intake, but they had to work quite hard at it. Some volunteers could maintain their new weight gain only with difficulty. If they subsequently reduced their food intake, their weight fell rapidly. Some had great difficulty in gaining even a slight increase in weight.

There was one especially interesting discovery. One man succeeded in doubling his body fat by overeating to the extent of a food intake of 7,000 calories a day over about 200 days. Within 100 days of returning to a diet of a little over 1,000 calories a day, his body weight had returned to normal. Interestingly enough, he had already lost about half of his increased body weight after ten days or so on a 3,000 calorie diet.

This experiment does answer some of the awkward questions asked about Mr Constant Weight and Mrs Fatten Easily. First of all they do exist. Second, even in Mrs Fatten Easily, there is a sort of weight gain/metabolic rate system that cuts in at a certain level of weight gain in *otherwise fit, overweight people*. Perhaps the best news to come out of this interesting experiment is that doctors and nutritionists must now believe the patient who says, 'Doctor, I don't really eat all that much and yet I gain weight'. They must also believe the equally worried person who says, 'There must be something wrong with me. I can't put on any weight, however much I eat'.

Spin-offs from this Vermont prison study produced some new, very technical knowledge on the subject of obesity, an area for biological debate. It also demonstrated that a few of our well-loved theories on obesity and slimming are based on somewhat shaky foundations. Most people associate obesity with physical sluggishness and lack of activity has, for many a day, been believed a cause of obesity. The Vermont study suggests, however, that we may have got it all the wrong way round. As the prisoners became heavier they *responded by being less active.*

In many of our diets we try to build in anti-hunger factors in the form of bulky food and bulk-type slimming aids. In the prison study, some men, eating enormous amounts of food (up to 10,000 calories a day), reported feeling hungry towards the end of the afternoon or even during the whole day. Clearly, the volume of food taken has little effect on appetite.

Many obese people worry about the fat levels in their blood and this has raised the spectre of the fat man eating his way to a heart attack. The Vermont survey showed no relationship between obesity and changes in blood fats (lipids) although, as we will see later, there is some association between overweight and heart disease.

A new and practical tip emerges from this experimental study. One factor seemed to help the fattened-up volunteers maintain their acquired obesity. This was enhanced appetite late in the day; a large evening intake of food at a time of reduced activity. This clearly conserves fuel and keeps the fat in place.

Nutritional experts and medical scientists are still trying to find a basic defect in Mrs Fatten Easily. Theories come and go with relentless regularity. At one time, it was mistakenly believed that the 'fatten easilies' had a basic metabolic defect, blamed, for many years, on a breakdown of pyruvic acid usage in the body. Nowadays, more attention is being paid to insulin and growth hormone studies. In all probability, however, no quick and happy solution will be found. More likely, the ability to fatten easily is an inborn trait—a variation in the human frame, with its roots in evolution rather than abnormality. Mrs Fatten Easily is at a biological advantage during times of famine. Perhaps, if she had not existed, the human race may have died out many years ago and we would not be here to worry about dieting.

How many ways to diet?

Broadly speaking, there are two ways to diet—balanced diets and unbalanced diets. It is extraordinary how quickly value judgments and evangelical ideas creep in, once you get to grips with dieting. I can almost hear people saying,

'Who wants to be *unbalanced* or even *off balance,* particularly with reference to something so close to life as food?' I would give unqualified approval to such critics, were it not for one thing. The basic reasoning behind the ideas of a balanced diet are, if not obscure, then at least slightly unrealistic in many ways.

Balanced diets

A word of explanation is necessary. The idea of balance in a diet assumes just the loss of fat and no other physiological alteration. In other words, no body protein (muscle tissue) is lost. Just enough carbohydrate is allowed to stop the phenomenon of ketosis occurring. (Ketosis, as explained in Chapter I, is a condition which occurs because there is an acute lack of carbo-hydrate in the diet. Fat then cannot entirely be converted into energy and water and so it gets 'stuck' at an incomplete metabolic stage.) It is assumed that, with a balanced diet, everything in the nutritional garden is lovely and the person concerned can go on healthily dieting until the desired weight is reached. Unfortunately, in practice, the picture is not so rosy. The balance is only maintained if the dieter continues to expend energy at around the level built into the calorie deficit, which is, in turn, built into the diet. An occasional, extra energy spurt, such as a game of golf, tennis or squash, or even an extra long walk with the dog, will unbalance the diet to some extent. Also, any diet is *balanced* around Mr Averageman, whoever he is. The week of slim-ming meals given at the end of this chapter is an example of a balanced diet.

Perhaps the really unbalancing factor in the balanced diet is that weight reduction is very slow and 500-900 g (1-2 lb) a week weight-loss is the rule. Often, there is no perceptible drop in weight for about two weeks. This is not because the fat has not been lost, but because the body's water content becomes temporarily disturbed. If this is not understood, the diet may be abandoned as useless, before it has started. That makes it a totally unbalanced slimming aid by anybody's definition of the term.

Unbalanced diets

Unbalanced diets include every other form of dieting, from starvation to the zaniest diets invented. This category also contains some of the most effective and successful diets such as the high fat diet and some high protein diets, so it could be said that the most unbalanced thing about them is the favourable loss of weight the dieter notices when he or she stands on the bathroom scales. Understandably, they make up the majority of the content of this book. The one you choose must depend on what sort of person you are, how quickly you want to slim, how fit you are, how rich you are and, in fact, all the basic prerequisites of embarking on a slimming regime.

What is in food

To understand diets and slimming you need a little specialized knowledge of nutrition, but not a lot. By the time you have finished reading this section (about five minutes) you will know enough on the subject.

Most fruit, vegetables and cereals, as they grow on the tree or in the field, are a mixture of the three basic elements of nutrition—protein, carbohydrate and fat. Animals, including birds and fish as well as ourselves, are mostly protein and fat. When dieticians talk about certain foods being *carbohydrates*, they usually mean *mostly carbohydrates*. Cakes are an example of these mostly carbohydrate foods. There are some foods which are pure carbohydrate, for example, sugar and syrup.

When dieticians talk about *fat*, meaning just fat alone, they are talking about butter, oils and cream. There are, however, many *high fat* foods, like cheese, fat meat and some fatty fishes, such as herring and salmon, that contain quite a lot of protein too. Cutting the fat off meat reduces its fat-content, but there is always a certain amount of fat left inside the meat fibres.

Protein in its pure form does not occur much in nature. Both plant and animal foods contain protein in variable amounts. Some vegetable foods, such as bread, are high in protein but animal foods (meat and fish) are our main sources of protein.

Foods also contain *roughage*. This refers to the indigestible content of food and the main constituent of roughage is fibre. However, in children and adults who experience over-frequent bowel motions, other items of their diet appear undigested in the motions and this forms part of the diet's roughage.

Most foods contain a considerable amount of *water*, except oils such as olive oil and cooking oil. Often the water content of food is responsible for its bulk and appearance, for example a prune is simply a plum minus its water.

All foods contain a variety of *mineral salts*—mostly calcium and sodium derivatives. Recently, mineral additives to food have been in vogue, but it is doubtful whether these are necessary in practice. The only mineral substance liable to be lacking in meat-free diets is iron, although many vegetarians manage to keep in good iron balance without supplementing their diet with iron preparations.

Vitamins are chemical substances which are present in natural foods. A deficiency of vitamins can cause various diseases or illnesses. There are two types, those that are oily or occur in certain fatty foods and those that are soluble in water. This distinction is practical as well as being scientific. The fatty vitamins A and D are stable substances during cooking and may be stored, to a certain extent, in the body. In other words, it takes a considerable length of time for a deficiency of Vitamins A and D to develop should the diet be deficient in them. The other vitamins, B and C, are unstable substances and are easily destroyed by cooking processes and, being water soluble, are lost from food when it is boiled in water. The body does not store them in the same way and so if they are persistently absent from the diet, deficiencies can develop quickly unless vitamin supplements are provided (see Chapter I).

Vitamins and minerals

Vitamin A	leafy vegetables, cheese, eggs
Vitamin D	fish (especially oily fish, such as herring)
Vitamin E	leafy vegetables, nuts, eggs
Vitamin K	green vegetables
Vitamin C	fruit (especially citrus) and vegetables
Vitamin B_1	grain, meat, poultry, fish, peas, beans
Vitamin B_2	cheese, eggs, meat, leafy vegetables
Vitamin B_{12}	meat, fish, eggs, cheese
Niacin	poultry, meat, fish, leafy vegetables
Pyridoxine (B_6)	meat
Pantothenic Acid	meat, fish, eggs, vegetables
Folic Acid	meat, fruit, eggs
Biotin	meat, eggs, peas, beans, nuts
Iron	meat, poultry, shellfish, eggs, nuts, green and leafy vegetables, fruit
Calcium	cheese, cottage cheese, salmon, shellfish, broccoli

Protein warning

Words of warning are very common in all diets, usually to prevent people from doing silly things. Often these dreadful warnings are superfluous, for people who embark on crazy diets usually come off them fairly quickly because they feel so bad. However, one thing must be remembered. We can survive, with difficulty, without any fat or carbohydrate in our diet, but we cannot live for very long without any protein.

Our bodies are constantly replacing protein, in our muscles, our blood corpuscles, our tissues everywhere, with vitally needed new protein. The only way we can build our vital proteins is by eating more protein. Science tells us that we all need a certain minimum protein intake per day, just to 'tick over'. Otherwise our muscles waste and we become weak. The amount we need is very small—about 1 g (0.035 oz) for every 1 kg (2.2 lb) of our body weight. The amount of actual food we need to produce this varies, because the protein content of different foods is very variable, but it is the basic element on which all sensible diets must be constructed.

Calories

When foods are looked at from the point of view of slimming, great emphasis is placed on carbohydrates and calories. Fattening diets always contain excessive amounts of carbohydrates. Therefore, one way to stop gaining or to lose weight is to reduce the amount of carbohydrate consumed. The part that calories alone play in slimming is not fully understood. Meals with a high calorie content can fatten, if their calorie content comes from carbohydrate, or if high quantities of fat (and protein) are taken with enough carbohydrate to make them fattening. Exactly what is enough carbohydrate in this context is the big debatable and variable question. It seems to be possible to eat lots of calories, say in the form of fat (see Chapter V) and lose weight, if there is virtually no carbohydrate in the meal as well. Equally, it is also possible to lose weight while eating almost anything, if you reduce your total calorie intake enough so that your body is using more calories than you are taking in.

What is in food, therefore, is very important. From the practical point of view, food has to be looked at in two ways —how much carbohydrate and how many calories, although the latter is not important if you are on a high fat diet.

Calorie and carbohydrate charts

Calorie charts for foods have been designed by scientists, who have worked out the calorific values of foods from the point of view of the energy they give out, i.e. the total energy content. The carbohydrate and calorie charts that follow give a rough and ready guide. However, doctors have taken certain *portions* of food with the same calorific value and found that, due to the way in which the food is digested and absorbed, there are wide energy intake variations in the 'equivalent' portions.

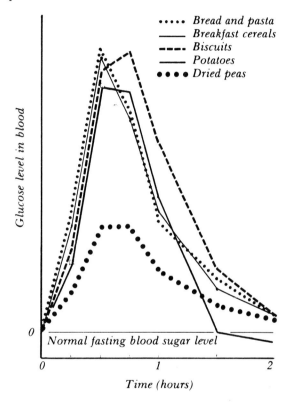

This graph shows the change in the concentration of glucose in the blood after eating 50-g (1¾-oz) carbohydrate portions of bread and pasta, breakfast cereals, biscuits, potatoes and dried peas. There is a wide difference in the way in which the blood glucose level rises between the different types of carbohydrates eaten. It is unrealistic to assume that all carbohydrates will be absorbed by the body in the same amounts. This graph shows that the amount of sugar absorbed by the body from dried peas is far lower than from the same quantity of bread, breakfast cereals and biscuits.

Fruit

Fruit is generally regarded as the slimmer's friend, but, if you are working out a diet with either calorie- or carbohydrate-restriction in mind, look carefully at your chosen fruit in the chart before you eat. For example, bananas are very similar to potatoes in this context and an egg matches half a grapefruit, with calories in mind. Knowing particularly the carbohydrate and calorie values helps you to introduce variety into the fruit content of your diet, without ruining its slimming potential. Fibre values give us an idea of how filling the fruit is. Notice how processing reduces fibre and therefore makes fruit less filling.

Contents per 100 g (3½ oz) edible portion (unless otherwise stated)	Carbo-hydrates		Calories
	gTotal	gFibre	kcal
Apples			
(sweet), fresh	15.0	0.9	58
1 apple 6 cm (2½ in) diameter	20.0	1.2	77
dried	73.6	4.0	281
Apple juice	13	–	47
Apple sauce, sweetened	19.7	0.6	72
Apricots			
fresh	12.9	0.6	51
1 apricot, medium	4.3	0.2	18
canned, sweetened	21.4	0.4	80
dried	66.9	3.2	262
Avocado	5.1	1.8	245
Bananas			
fresh	23.0	0.6	89
1 banana, 15 cm (6 in)	23.0	0.6	89
Blackberries			
fresh	12.5	4.2	57
canned, sweetened	22.8	2.9	86
Cherries	14.6	0.5	60
Cranberries	11.3	1.4	48
Cranberry sauce	51.4	0.4	188
Currants			
red, fresh	13.6	4.0	55
black, fresh	16.1	5.7	62
Dates, dried	75.4	2.4	284
Figs			
fresh	16.1	1.4	65
dried	68.4	5.8	258
Fruit cocktail, canned	18.6	0.4	70
Gooseberries	9.7	1.9	39
Grapes	16.7	0.5	66
Grape juice	18.2	–	67
Grapefruit			
fresh	9.8	0.5	39
½ grapefruit 16 cm (4¼ in) diameter	18.4	0.9	73
canned, sweetened	19.1	0.2	72
Grapefruit juice	9.2	0.1	36
Lemons			
fresh	8.7	0.9	32
1 lemon 5 cm (2 in) diameter	5.4	0.6	21

Contents per 100 g (3½ oz) edible portion (unless otherwise stated)	Carbo-hydrates g Total	g Fibre	Calories kcal
Lemon juice	7.7	-	24
Lime juice	8.3		24
Melon			
cantaloupe	4.6	0.6	20
water	6.9	0.6	28
Olives, green	4.0	1.2	132
Oranges			
fresh	11.2	0.6	45
1 orange 8 cm (3 in) diameter	17.5	0.9	70
Orange juice, fresh	12.9	0.1	49
Peaches			
fresh	11.8	0.6	46
canned, sweetened	18.2	0.4	68
dried	69.4	3.5	265
Pears			
fresh	15.5	1.5	61
1 pear 6 cm (2½ in) diameter	23.4	2.3	92
canned, sweetened	18.4	0.8	68
Pineapple			
fresh	12.2	0.5	47
canned, sweetened	21.1	0.3	78
Pineapple juice, canned	13.0	0.1	49
Plums			
fresh	12.9	0.5	50
1 plum 5 cm (2 in) diameter	7.4	0.3	29
canned, sweetened	20.4	0.3	76
Prunes, uncooked	71.0	1.6	268
Quinces	14.9	2.4	57
Raisins	71.2	6.8	268
Raspberries			
fresh	13.8	4.7	57
canned, sweetened	28.	-	107
Raspberry juice	11	trace	40
Strawberries			
fresh	8.3	1.4	37
canned, sweetened	28	0.7	104
Tangerines	10.9	1.0	44

Nuts

Nuts may not be as calorific as they look in the tables. Unless they are very scrupulously and completely chewed up, quite a large proportion goes through the bowel unchanged.

Contents per 100 g (3½ oz) edible portion (unless otherwise stated)	Carbo-hydrates g Total	g Fibre	Calories kcal
Almonds	19.6	2.0	640
Brazil nuts	11	2.1	695
Chestnuts			
fresh	45.6	1.3	213
dried	79	2.5	380
Coconuts			
fresh	12.8	3.3	351
dried	53.2	4.1	579
Hazel nuts	18	3.4	671
Peanuts	23.4	3.3	546
Walnuts	15.6	2.1	702

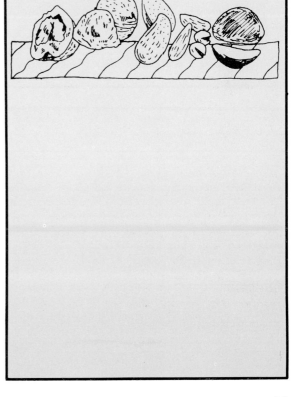

Vegetables

As in the case of fruit, look for calorie and carbohydrate traps—and bonuses. Although in most cases the values are reliable, modern research has shown that the amount of *available* carbohydrate in some vegetables is less than the tables show. This is probably due to the fact that enzymes, by means of which we digest food, do not break down all food completely. Dried peas are an example of this. As the tables show, dried peas have high carbohydrate and calorie scores. However, as shown in the glucose concentration graph, tests have proved that the amount of glucose (sugar) that the body extracts from them is much less than from a similar weight of bread, pasta and potatoes. Fibre rich foods again have good value as fillers but cooking these foods quickly 'loses' fibre.

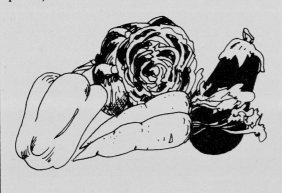

Contents per 100 g (3½ oz) edible portion (unless otherwise stated)	Carbo-hydrates		Calories
	g Total	g Fibre	kcal
Artichokes, Jerusalem	10.6	2.7	49
Asparagus			
fresh	4.1	0.8	21
canned	2.9	0.5	18
Aubergine	5.5	0.9	24
Beans			
green, fresh	7.7	1.4	41
canned	4.7	0.5	26
broad, fresh	23.5	1.5	128
canned	18.3	2.0	95
kidney	61.6	4.0	338
Beetroot	9.6	0.9	42
Broccoli	5.5	1.3	29
Brussels sprouts	8.7	1.2	47
Cabbage			
red	5.9	1.1	26
white	5.7	1.5	25
Carrots			
fresh	9.1	1.0	40
1 carrot 15 cm (6 in) long	4.5	0.5	20
canned	6.4	0.8	30
Cauliflower	4.9	0.9	25
Celery, stalk	8.8	-	45
Chicory	3.7	0.6	16
Courgettes	3.6	0.6	17
Cucumbers			
fresh	3.0	0.6	13
1 medium cucumber	8.7	1.7	38

Cereals

Note the calorie/carbohydrate advantages of using wholemeal flour in diets. Proprietary breakfast foods are not included in this list. Many of these are highly calorific. For example, cornflakes contain 385 calories per 100 g. Crispbreads contain 345 calories per 100 g, but, as only one or two slices are consumed, they help in most slimming breakfasts.

Many basic foods containing cereals are difficult to define in terms of carbohydrate or calories, as recipes alter matters. Most cakes contain about 370 calories per 100 g, biscuits and cookies about 440 calories per 100 g, suet puddings 370 calories per 100 g and tapioca 360 calories per 100 g. Rice pudding is quite low in calories at about 140 calories per 100 g, and so are blancmange at 120 calories per 100 g, and bread and butter pudding at 162 calories per 100 g. It is quite easy to consume 100 g of biscuits or cookies and they spoil many calorie diets. Even biscuits, cookies and crackers which do not 'look' fattening are high in calories—cream crackers 450 calories per 100 g, digestives 480 calories per 100 g, general plain mixed 435 calories per 100 g and sweet 555 calories per 100 g.

Contents per 100 g (3½ oz) edible portion (unless otherwise stated)	Carbohydrates g Total	g Fibre	Calories kcal	Contents per 100 g (3½ oz) edible portion (unless otherwise stated)	Carbohydrates g Total	g Fibre	Calories kcal
Fennel	6.4	-	27	Rhubarb	3.8	0.7	16
Garlic	29.3	1.1	129	Soya beans, dried	34.8	5.0	331
Horseradish	18.1	2.8	80	Spinach			
Kale	7.2	1.2	40	fresh	3.2	0.6	20
Kohlrabi, tubers	6.7	1.1	30	canned	3.0	0.7	20
Leeks	9.4	1.2	44	Sweetcorn			
Lentils, dried	59.5	3.7	337	fresh	20.5	0.8	92
Lettuce	2.8	0.6	15	canned, drained	20.2	1.1	85
Marrow	3.6	0.6	17	Tomatoes			
Mushrooms	3.7	0.9	22	fresh	4.0	0.6	19
Onions				1 tomato 6 cm (2½ in)			
fresh	10.3	0.8	45	diameter	6.0	0.9	29
1 onion 6 cm (2½ in)				canned	3.9	0.4	18
diameter	11.3	0.9	50	Tomato juice, canned	4.3	0.2	19
dried	80.2	4.5	347	Tomato ketchup	9.5	0.5	44
Parsley	9.0	1.8	50	Turnips			
Parsnips	18.2	2.2	78	fresh	7.1	1.1	32
Peas				greens	5.4	1.2	30
fresh	17.0	2.2	80	Watercress	3.3	0.5	18
canned	12.7	1.3	67	Yeast			
dried	61.7	1.2	345	baker's, compressed	13.0	0.3	79
Peppers, green	5.3	1.4	24	brewer's, dried	37.4	0.8	249
Potatoes							
fresh	19.1	0.4	83				
crisps	49.1	1.1	544				
dried	82.2	2.2	357				
Pumpkins	3.5	0.6	15				
Radishes	4.2	0.7	20				

Contents per 100 g (3½ oz) edible portion (unless otherwise stated)	Carbohydrates g Total	g Fibre	Calories kcal	Contents per 100 g (3½ oz) edible portion (unless otherwise stated)	Carbohydrates g Total	g Fibre	Calories kcal
Barley, pearl	76.5	0.8	346	white, unenriched	76.1	0.3	363
Bread				Oatflakes	67.6	1.4	387
rye	52.4	0.4	244	Pancakes	26.6	0.1	218
white, enriched	51.6	0.2	275	Pasta, unenriched, dry	73.2	0.4	381
toasted	59.0	0.2	313	Pastry, plain, unenriched	53.1	0.2	487
wholemeal	49.0	1.5	240	Popcorn, popped	76.7	2.2	386
Cornflour	87.0	0.1	362	Rice			
Flour				brown	77.7	0.6	360
rye, dark	73.1	2.0	325	white, cooked	26.2	0.1	119
self-raising, enriched	73.8	0.1	350	Semolina, wheat	76	-	362
soya bean, full fat	29.9	2.3	347	Spaghetti, unenriched, dry	76.5	0.4	376
medium fat	37.2	2.6	261	Tapioca, dry	86.4	0.1	360
wheat, whole	71.5	2.1	331	Wheatgerm	49.5	2.5	361

Meat and fish

The relatively high calorie content of meat compared with fish is interesting. Offal is usually lower in calories than other meat.

Contents per 100 g (3½ oz) edible portion (unless otherwise stated)	g Carbohydrates	Calories
		kcal
Meat, Poultry		
(raw unless otherwise stated)		
Bacon		
medium fat	trace	625
Beef, medium fat		
hamburger, cooked	0	365
rib roast, cooked	0	319
rump, cooked	0	378
sirloin	-	243
canned, corned	0	216
dried, salted	0	203
brains	0.8	120
heart	0.6	128
kidneys	0.9	141
liver	5.9	136
tongue	0.4	207
tripe	0	99
Calf (see also Veal)		
brains	0.8	122
heart	0.8	124
kidneys	0.8	132
liver	4.0	141
sweetbreads	0	111
Chicken		
grilling	0	151
roasting	0	200
canned	0	199
liver	2.6	141
Duck, medium fat	0	326
Goose, medium fat	0	354
liver	5.5	184

Contents per 100 g (3½ oz) edible portion (unless otherwise stated)	g Carbohydrates	Calories kcal	Contents per 100 g (3½ oz) edible portion (unless otherwise stated)	g Carbohydrates	Calories kcal
			Fish (raw unless otherwise stated)		
Ham			Carp	0	145
raw	0	345	Caviar, pressed	-	299
boiled	0	269	Clams	3.4	80
smoked, raw	0.3	389	Cod	0	74
canned, spiced	1.5	289	Crab, canned or cooked,		
Hare	0.2	103	meat only	1.3	103
Lamb, medium fat			Eel		
leg roast, cooked	0	274	fresh	0	285
rib chop, cooked	0	418	smoked	0.8	333
shoulder, cooked	0	342	Haddock	0	79
heart	0	124	Halibut	0	126
kidneys	0	105	Herring		
liver	0	136	fresh	0	243
Mutton, medium fat	0	187	smoked	0	211
Pork (see also Bacon and Ham)			Lobster		
cutlets	0	341	fresh	0.5	88
loin or chops, cooked	0	333	canned	0.4	92
ribs	0	351	Mackerel	0	188
brains	trace	126	Oysters	4.8	68
heart	0.4	117	Perch	0	86
kidneys	0.8	120	Pike	-	89
liver	1.7	134	Plaice	0	68
Rabbit	0	159	Salmon		
Sausages			fresh	0	208
beef	15.7	286	canned	0	173
frankfurter	2.7	256	Sardines		
pork	9.8	335	canned in oil	1.0	338
salami	-	524	drained	1.2	214
Turkey, medium fat	0.4	270	Scallops	3.4	77
Veal			Shrimps		
leg, raw	0	190	fresh	-	97
cutlet, cooked	0	219	canned	0.3	89
shoulder roast, cooked	0	228	Trout	0	101
stew meat, cooked	0	296	Tuna, canned	0	290
Venison	0	124			

Fat and dairy products

The very high calorific values for fats and oils is the reason for their exclusion, except in small quantities, from slimming diets, apart from high fat diets (see Chapter V), where special factors apply. Butter bought in individual portion packs is expensive but can help butter lovers. Frying food approximately doubles its calorie content, except in the case of potatoes, when it triples it.

Contents per 100 g (3½ oz) edible portion (unless otherwise stated)	g Carbohydrates	Calories kcal
Fats, Oils		
Butter	0.7	716
Cod-liver oil	0	901
Corn oil	0	883
Lard	0	901
Mayonnaise	3.0	708
Olive oil	0	883
Palm oil	0	883
Peanut butter	21.0	576
Peanut oil	0	883
Soya bean oil	0	883
Sunflower oil	0	883
Dairy products, Eggs		
Butter, see under Fats, above		
Cheese		
Camembert	1.8	287
Cheddar	2.1	398
Cottage	2.7	86
Cream	2.1	374
Emmenthal	3.4	398

Contents per 100 g (3½ oz) edible portion (unless otherwise stated)	g Carbohydrates	Calories kcal
Parmesan	2.9	393
Roquefort	1.8	378
Cream, double	2.9	288
Eggs		
whole, raw	0.7	162
Egg white, raw	0.8	51
Egg yolk, raw	0.7	361
1 egg, medium	0.4	77
1 egg white, medium	0.3	16
1 egg yolk, medium	0.1	61
Egg powder	2.5	604
Milk (cow's)		
pasteurized, whole	4.6	64
buttermilk, cultured	4.0	35
condensed (sweetened)	54.8	320
canned, evaporated (unsweetened)	9.9	138
dried, whole	38.0	492
non-fat	52.0	362

Confectionery and jams

There are no safe foods for slimmers here.

Contents per 100 g (3½ oz) edible portion (unless otherwise stated)	Carbo-hydrates Total g	Fibre g	Calories kcal
Caramel	78.0	–	416
Chocolate			
sweetened, milk	55.7	0.5	509
plain	62.7	1.4	471
Cocoa, dry powder	43.6	5.7	299
Dextrose, anhydrous	99.5	0	385
Honey	79.5	–	294
Jams	70.8	0.6	278
Sugar			
brown	96	–	372
cane or beet, white	99.5	0	385
Treacle	60.0	–	232

Drinks

Tea and coffee, without milk or sugar, are virtually calorie- and carbohydrate-free. However, 100 g of milk (five cups of tea or coffee) will add 66 calories and the average lump of sugar equals 18 calories. Unsweetened, slim-line or diet soda drinks are virtually calorie-free, but all alcoholic drinks are calorific. 'Crazy' dieting is to feel so deprived that you give up potatoes, at about 80 calories per 100 g, and substitute two large glasses of gin, at 245 calories! Many alcohol drinkers unconsciously consume huge quantities of calories. An apparently modest half-bottle of wine may well provide around 300 calories.

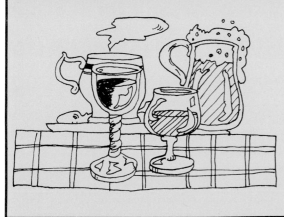

Contents per 100 g (3½ oz) edible portion (unless otherwise stated)	Calories kcal
Non-alcoholic	
Carbonated soft drinks	39
Cola drinks	41
Coffee (unsweetened)	5
Tea (unsweetened)	2
Alcoholic	
Beer 275 ml (½ pint)	88
Brandy	262
Gin	245
Port wine	136
Rum	245
Sherry	
dry	120
sweet	135
Whisky	245
Wine	
dry	60
sweet	100

Low-calorie foods

Incredibly, there are some foods which are so low in carbohydrates that they shine in the eyes of all wise dieters. They include artichokes (globe), asparagus and French beans, runner beans, cabbage/savoy, celery, chicory, cucumber, marrow and courgettes, mushrooms, oysters, unsweetened stewed rhubarb, sea-kale and spring greens.

Foods to avoid

Diets do not often mention the calorie content of the following foods.

Beefburger	246 calories per 100 g
Steak and kidney pudding	500 calories per 100 g
Sausage roll	500 calories per 100 g
Pizza	359 calories per 100 g
Pasta	400 calories per 100 g
Baked jam roll	450 calories per 100 g
Syrup sponge pudding	360 calories per 100 g
Slice of chocolate cake or flan	500 calories per 100 g
Chocolates	550 calories per 100 g

These are expensive ways to spend a calorie ration.

(Tables extracted from *Documenta Geigy Scientific Tables,* 7th edition. Courtesy CIBA- GEIGY Limited, Basle, Switzerland.)

Beef extract diet

There is an attraction about a very simple diet for people who have not the time to plan themselves an elaborate change of their eating patterns. The Bovril slimming diet has been worked out around simple cooking and economy. It is a 1,500 calorie diet and is suitable for those who do not have too much weight to shed. It is also suitable for those slimmers who have lost weight on either the Basic I or II low carbohydrate diets (see Chapter IV) and who now need to follow a less strict diet.

	MONDAY		TUESDAY		WEDNESDAY		
BREAKFAST		Calories		Calories		Calories	
	Orange juice	60	Half grapefruit	15	Fruit juice	60	
	1 slice of bacon	169	1 poached egg	90	125 g (4 oz) grilled		
	2 grilled tomatoes	20	1 piece of toast	51	kipper	124	
	1 piece of toast	51	1 pat of butter	55	1 slice of bread	51	
	1 pat of butter	55			1 pat of butter	55	
LUNCH	1 mug hot Bovril	17	75 g (3 oz) canned		1 mug hot Bovril	17	
	1 crispbread spread		salmon	117	2 tomatoes	20	
	with Bovril	42	Cucumber	0	50 g (2 oz) cottage		
	125 g (4 oz) lean ham	250	2 slices of bread	102	cheese	60	
	Lettuce	0	2 pats of butter	112	2 slices of lean ham	125	
	1 apple	40	1 orange	40	Cucumber and lettuce	0	
					1 pear	35	
DINNER	1 grilled lamb chop	435	125 g (4 oz) lean,		125 g (4 oz) cold		
	125 g (4 oz) green		roast lamb	330	lean lamb	330	
	vegetables	20	125 g (4 oz) cauliflower		1 small, baked potato	45	
	125 g (4 oz) carrots	20	with 25 g (1 oz)		1 pat of butter	55	
	1 small, boiled potato	45	grated Edam cheese	88	125 g (4 oz) green		
	1 slice of melon	15	1 small, boiled potato	45	vegetables	20	
	150 ml (5 fl oz) plain		125 g (4 oz) carrots	20	Canned or fresh celery		
	yogurt	75	1 apple	40	braised in Bovril	8	
					1 baked apple	65	
	TOTAL	1314	TOTAL	1105	TOTAL	1070	

* Total daily ration of milk = 275 ml (½ pint).
* Spread Bovril on bread and crispbread instead of butter.
* Drink a mug of hot Bovril instead of milky bedtime drinks.
* Total calorie allowance per day, including milk ration = 1,500 calories.

THURSDAY	Calories	FRIDAY	Calories	SATURDAY	Calories	SUNDAY	Calories
Half grapefruit	15	Half grapefruit	15	Fruit juice	60	Half grapefruit	15
1 slice of bacon	169	1 boiled egg	90	1 large, grilled beef		40 g (1½ oz) Edam cheese	
1 grilled tomato	10	1 crispbread	26	sausage	155	grilled on 1 piece	
1 slice of bread	51	½ pat of butter	28	50 g (2 oz) grilled		of toast	183
1 pat of butter	55			mushrooms	4		
				1 slice of bread	51		
				1 pat of butter	55		
125 g (4 oz) corned		125 g (4 oz) cold		1 mug hot Bovril	17	1 mug hot Bovril	17
beef	260	tongue	335	2 crispbreads	52	1 crispbread spread	
125 g (4 oz) cucumber	10	2 tomatoes	20	25 g (1 oz) liver		with Bovril	42
2 slices of bread		50 g (2 oz)		sausage	92	125 g (4 oz) tongue	335
spread with Bovril	134	Camembert cheese	175	1 tomato	10	2 tomatoes	20
150 ml (5 fl oz) plain		2 crispbreads	52	125 g (4 oz) cottage		1 orange	40
yogurt	75	1 pat of butter	55	cheese	120		
		1 apple	40	1 celery stalk	5		
				1 slice of bread	51		
175 g (6 oz) poached,		125 g (4 oz) lambs' liver		1 grilled, lean pork		1 slice of grilled	
smoked haddock	120	and 1 slice of bacon		chop	510	bacon	169
1 poached egg	90	casseroled in		1 slice of pineapple	45	1 grilled sausage	155
125 g (4 oz) green		Bovril	240	125 g (4 oz) green		1 grilled tomato	10
vegetables	20	125 g (4 oz) green		vegetables	20	1 fried egg	135
2 small, boiled		beans	10	75 g (3 oz) sweetcorn	75	1 slice of bread	
potatoes	90	125 g (4 oz) carrots	20	1 grilled tomato	10	spread with Bovril	67
2 slices of canned		2 small, boiled		1 baked apple	65	50 g (2 oz) Camembert	
pineapple, drained	90	potatoes	90			cheese	175
Orange juice	60	1 orange	40			1 celery stalk	5
TOTAL	**1249**	**TOTAL**	**1236**	**TOTAL**	**1397**	**TOTAL**	**1368**

(Based on *The Bovril Slimming Diet*)

41

Week of slimming meals

The diet which follows is based on calorie content. Protein, carbohydrates and fat are balanced in the correct proportions. Average-sized portions, unless specified in the diet, can be varied depending on whether or not the person is doing a lot of muscular work, in which case larger portions are allowed, or sedentary work, in which case portions must be restricted. Meat and fish portions are 100 g (3½ oz) unless specified. Weight-loss depends on the amount of exercise taken (see Chapter XII) and you should lose between 225-500 g (8 oz-1 lb) per week.

	MONDAY	TUESDAY	WEDNESDAY	
BREAKFAST	Unsweetened fruit juice Scrambled eggs 1 piece of toast with butter Tea or coffee (no sugar)	Grapefruit Kidneys and bacon 1 piece of toast with butter Tea or coffee (no sugar)	22 g (¾ oz) cornflakes with milk but no sugar Bacon and egg 1 piece of toast with butter Tea or coffee (no sugar)	
MID-MORNING	Tea or coffee (no sugar)	Tea or coffee (no sugar)	Tea or coffee (no sugar)	
LUNCH	Vegetable soup Roast chicken Brussels sprouts, small helping buttered carrots 1 or 2 small potatoes Stewed apple with cream	Frankfurters Grilled tomatoes, frozen beans or green salad Small helping rice pudding (sweetened with saccharine) Grapes (small portion)	Tomato juice Grilled steak, 1 or 2 small potatoes 50 g (2 oz) mushrooms Green salad (oil and vinegar dressing) Egg custard (sweetened with saccharine)	
AFTERNOON	Tea or coffee (no sugar)	Tea or coffee (no sugar)	Tea or coffee (no sugar)	
DINNER	75 g (3 oz) cheese, hard-boiled egg Mixed salad (oil and vinegar dressing) 1 slice of bread and butter Plain yogurt without sugar	Chicken or plain omelet Spinach Cheese, with starch-reduced crispbread and butter Fresh fruit	Smoked haddock Frozen peas 1 slice of bread and butter Fresh orange	
NIGHTCAP	Milk, or hot meat or vegetable extract, or lemon juice	Milk, or hot meat or vegetable extract, or lemon juice	Milk, or hot meat or vegetable extract, or lemon juice	
DAILY RATION	275 ml (½ pint) milk	275 ml (½ pint) milk	275 ml (½ pint) milk	

THURSDAY	FRIDAY	SATURDAY	SUNDAY
Porridge with salt and milk (no sugar) Grilled bacon and tomatoes 1 slice of bread and butter Tea or coffee (no sugar)	Tomato juice Bacon and egg 1 piece of toast with butter Tea or coffee (no sugar)	Grapefruit Grilled kippers 1 slice of bread and butter Tea or coffee (no sugar)	Unsweetened fruit juice Scrambled eggs 1 piece of toast with butter Tea or coffee (no sugar)
Tea or coffee (no sugar)	Tea or coffee (no sugar)	Tea or coffee (no sugar)	Tea or coffee (no sugar)
Grilled chops (1 only if large) Leeks, small helping peas, 1 baked potato Stewed rhubarb with cream or evaporated milk (unsweetened)	Beef stew with carrots and onions Brussels sprouts Stewed gooseberries or blackcurrants (use saccharine) and cream	Roast lamb Cauliflower (no sauce) and carrots, or small potatoes Fresh fruit salad with cream	Steak and kidney pie (small piece of pastry) Cabbage and carrots Stewed pears (sweetened with saccharine) with cream or evaporated milk (unsweetened)
Tea or coffee (no sugar)	Tea or coffee (no sugar)	Tea or coffee (no sugar)	Tea or coffee (no sugar)
Cold meat and hard-boiled egg Mixed salad (oil and vinegar dressing) 1 slice of bread and butter Plain yogurt without sugar	Vegetable soup Grilled fish or 125 g (4 oz) cheese, with crispbread and butter Fresh fruit	Liver, bacon and mushrooms Grilled tomatoes Cheese with crispbread and butter	Grilled fish fingers, or plaice Grilled tomatoes Small helping frozen peas Fresh fruit
Milk, or hot meat or vegetable extract, or lemon juice	Milk, or hot meat or vegetable extract, or lemon juice	Milk, or hot meat or vegetable extract, or lemon juice	Milk, or hot meat or vegetable extract, or lemon juice
275 ml (½ pint) milk	275 ml (½ pint) milk	275 ml (½ pint) milk	275 ml (½ pint) milk

(Courtesy of *Slim and Enjoy It* by Dennis Craddock, a Family Doctor British Medical Association booklet)

CHAPTER IV

Low carbohydrate dieting

Low carbohydrate diets are thought by many eminent nutritionists to be the most suitable for weight control and for general nutritional health and well-being. It is important for the slimmer to get away from junk foods, rich in sugar, and to concentrate on natural foods, high in nutrients.

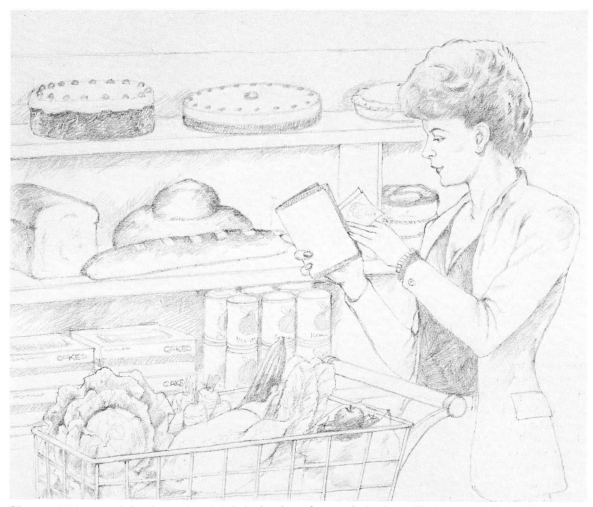

Chapter III has explained exactly what is in food including the number of calories it contains. The diet which follows is tailor-made for carbohydrate calorie counters and those who decide that a low carbohydrate diet is the easiest way for them to lose weight. If you choose this type of diet, you are in good company, for many eminent nutritionists believe that low carbohydrate diets are the most suitable, not only for weight control, but for general nutritional health and well-being.

The scientific fans of low carbohydrate diets argue that, as we move further away from the mode of life adopted over the millions of years since Man came down from the trees to live on the land, we greatly increase the chances that dietary changes will have ill effects on our frame. This is, of course, particularly the case when we remember that, in order to be really successful, dieting means altering patterns of food intake for a very long time. This is especially so in the case of

low carbohydrate dieting. This diet really means changing your way of eating for the rest of your life and, of course, staying slim.

Back to nature

Low carbohydrate dieting is pleasantly close to nature and nature cures are understandably back in fashion, for one very good reason—they work! This does not mean that you must spend all the weekly food budget at the health-food shop and live on sesame seeds, compost-grown vegetables, unsprayed apples and stone-ground wheat. All it means is that we are likely to be healthier and slimmer if we eat the sorts of foods eaten by our Neolithic ancestors whenever possible. We can still take advantage of the bonuses provided by modern technology—freezing, canning and other forms of food preservation.

The big and important message in low

carbohydrate dieting in the modern world is to get as far away from 'made-up' and 'junk' foods as we possibly can. These are rich in sugars and sugars are what modern Man consumes in quantities far in excess of his forebears. There is evidence that the human animal is not naturally adapted to consume the quantites of sugars and made-up foods, such as mass-produced bread, cakes and pastas, that we eat in the modern world. Because of this lack of adaptation, contemporary patterns of eating may well take us slowly but relentlessly down a path towards a whole host of diseases in which obesity seems to play a causative part.

Think nutrient not energy

The scientific enthusiasts for low carbohydrate diets quite rightly point out their intrinsic nutritional advantages, as well as dwelling on the dangers inherent in certain modern eating practices. One of the greatest and most phoney advertising 'sells' of our age is that certain foods provide 'energy'. A multitude of advertisements concentrates on selling manufactured products designed, they claim, to 'fill the energy gap' or to set the whole family up with energy as quickly as you can open the packet, turn back the plastic covering, and usually add the sugar or syrup (more energy). This led John Yudkin, Emeritus Professor of Nutrition, University of London, to stress what he called the low energy-high nutrient principle.

The table (right) shows the high nutrient content of certain foods low in carbohydrates compared with foods rich in carbohydrates.

Getting away from the *energy* concept of food, so lovingly and carefully implanted in our minds by manufacturers and advertisers, and concentrating on high *nutrient* food is the quick and easy template for all low carbohydrate diets. There are very important no-go areas in this sort of diet, which include all sugars and sugary substances.

Restrict carbohydrate intake

The principle of the diet involves restricting the total carbohydrate intake to 60-70 g (2-2½ oz) per day. Alcohol in the diet is included in the carbohydrate count. In practice, this means the avoidance of foods and drinks containing added sugar and using the tables and charts to restrict food containing carbohydrates, to maintain the magic figure of 60-70 g (2-2½ oz) per day. Such a diet is nutritionally sound for all adults and

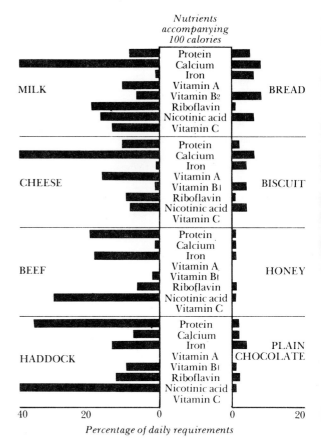

Nutrients accompanying 100 calories

Percentage of daily requirements

High nutrient content of foods low in carbohydrates and low nutrient content of foods rich in carbohydrates

children. Because it does not restrict the protein or fat taken, it usually contains all the vitamins and minerals necessary to good health.

Carbohydrates and seduction

The low carbohydrate diet has an element of puritanism if not asceticism about it, which the carbohydrate addict will find hard to resist. Many of the pastry cook's greatest and most seductive products finish up on the discard pile when the carbohydrates are being counted. Many 'high energy' foods are also highly palatable and so to eat just one bite and no more is virtually impossible. A 50-calorie portion of a choice gateau is about as pleasurable to a carbohydrate fancier as a small gin is to an alcoholic.

People who fall for the 'energy-gap' confidence trick of the confectioner are not really after the 'energy', they are after the taste. What goes for 'energy' foods and snacks is also true of certain similar drinks. However, besides the matter of taste, habituation of the drugs they contain is also a consideration. Sugarless black coffee and tea are virtually calorie-free, but a real tea or coffee addict may consume about 600 ml (1 pint) of milk a day in cups of tea or coffee, without noticing, in an otherwise well constructed, low carbohydrate, calorie controlled diet. Cola drinks contain caffeine, which is as addictive as that in tea and coffee, but in this case you have no chance to leave the sugar out. Beers that 'refresh' or provide the 'energy' that the hard worker needs morning, noon and night, are loaded with calories and alcohol, which is really just another low nutrient carbohydrate in disguise.

Full not fat

Although it is hard to judge satiety in a strictly objective way, it is possible to make a few, fairly accurate guesses. If we pitch a good, average, low carbohydrate reducing diet at 1,600 calories, it will contain 70 g (2½ oz) of carbohydrate, 100 g (3½ oz) of protein and 100 g (3½ oz) of fat and will leave Mr and Mrs Average doing the average amount of work, feeling averagely satisfied. A lot of averages you say? Yes, I agree, but the same average people on the same routine, but eating without carbohydrate control, will take about 250 g (8¾ oz) of carbohydrate to feel averagely satisfied. This gives 2,300 calories. So you can see where that stored weight comes from.

Different ways to diet

Two rather separate, if related, dietary principles are included in our low carbohydrate calorie counting diet review. Basic I and Basic II diets are very strictly, calorie controlled diets in which the body is forced to use up its own fat stores. There is no other biological possibility and the diet always works. Weight-loss inevitably results from following these diets, even if it is rather slow to begin. The diets are finely balanced to succeed in all cases of obesity—even the most refractory ones—provided that the dieter has the patience and will-power to persevere.

Unit eating, devised by Professor Yudkin, is something of a dietary package deal and, like many holiday package deals, is very good value. It concentrates on dieting by carbohydrate control without being too fussy over total calories. It is probably fair to say that there is not the same certainty about weight-loss with Unit dieting as there is with Basic I and Basic II diets. However, it works very well for some dieters and it could be that there are differing groups of people who respond best to differing dietary techniques.

Pre-diet regimes

One of the disadvantages of low carbohydrate, calorie control is that weight is lost slowly. At times, it may appear that no weight is lost at all, due to fluid retention within the body or constipation, if a large volume of food has been the habit. One way around this less than exciting beginning to a brand new and therapeutic resolution is to start with a three-day fast or a three-day fruit diet. For practical purposes, this has to coincide with a long weekend, when you have nothing to do but lie around reading novels, listening to the radio and watching television. You need to rest while you are on a three-day fast or a 'blitz start'.

Both these pre-diet regimes provide a four-fold bonus. They mark the beginning of dieting with a very definite 'event' and thus provide a good psychological marker. Second, they demonstrate, by the scales, that dieting works. Third, they reduce the appetite. Finally, they make the diet that follows seem much more adequate and satisfying and and so help avoid hunger.

During a three-day fast, unsweetened drinks are allowed in unlimited quantities. The body will lose about 175 g (6 oz) of its muscle tissue per day on this regime, and so a feeling of muscular 'weakness' will be experienced.

A less harsh and traumatic, zip-start to a diet is a one- to three-day fruit diet. Four portions of any of the following are allowed per day, together with unlimited black coffee and milkless tea. Lettuce, cucumber, watercress and mustard and cress can also be eaten. The fruit portions are carefully matched to prevent ketosis, a condition resulting from an acute lack of carbohydrate (see Chapter I), and reduce body protein loss.

Fruit portions
1 Orange juice 110 ml (4 fl oz) with 15 g (½ oz) sugar.
2 Pineapple juice 175 ml (6 fl oz).
3 Lemon juice 225 ml (8 fl oz) with 15 g (½ oz) sugar.
4 Tomato juice 110 ml (4 fl oz) plus 1 pear and 1 orange.
5 Melon 175 g (6 oz) with 15 g (½ oz) sugar.
6 Grapes 75 g (3 oz) plus plums 125 g (4 oz).

Basic I diet

Low carbohydrate, low calorie diet

	Carbohydrates g	Calories kcal
BREAKFAST		
Tea with lemon (or milk allowance)	—	—
2 eggs, boiled	—	154
25 g (1 oz) bread	15	78
LUNCH		
75 g (3 oz) lean meat	—	235
75 g (3 oz) potatoes	15	70
Low-calorie green vegetables	—	20
TEA		
Tea with lemon (or milk allowance)	—	—
25 g (1 oz) bread	15	78
Lettuce and medium-sized tomato	—	10
DINNER		
150 g (5 oz) plaice or other white fish, steamed	—	97
50 g (2 oz) potatoes, boiled	10	47
125 g (4 oz) orange	10	51
110 ml (4 fl oz) milk, to be taken throughout the day	5	70
TOTAL	**70**	**910**

Basic II diet

Low carbohydrate, low calorie diet

	Carbohydrates g	Calories kcal
BREAKFAST		
Tea with lemon	—	—
25 g (1 oz) bread	15	78
125 g (4 oz) orange	10	51
MID-MORNING		
Unsweetened lemonade or yeast extract	—	—
Medium-sized tomato and lettuce	—	10
Bran biscuit	—	—
125 g (4 oz) apple	15	66
LUNCH		
175 g (6 oz) lean meat	—	450
Low-calorie green vegetables	—	20
Food valueless jelly	—	—
TEA		
Tea with lemon	—	—
25 g (1 oz) bread	15	78
Medium-sized tomato and lettuce	—	10
DINNER		
175 g (6 oz) white fish, steamed	—	116
50 g (2 oz) potatoes	10	47
Low-calorie green vegetables	—	20
TOTAL	**65**	**946**

Basic I and Basic II diets

Basic I diet will produce a guaranteed weight-loss of 500-900 g (1-2 lb) a week. It allocates about 900 calories per day. It is advisable to supplement such a diet with vitamins.

Even on this fairly strict diet there is often a delay of 10-14 days before any weight-loss becomes evident on the scales. This may be obviated by excluding salt from the diet. This 'scales-lag' does not reflect what your diet is really doing for you—using up your fat stores, which is the real name of the game.

Basic II diet is a stricter low carbohydrate diet, which will give a very effective weight-loss, while allowing for two fairly substantial meals per day.

Both Basic I and Basic II diets have been worked out for mainly sedentary people but they can be scaled-up to match the calorie requirements of more active workers. Clearly, high energy expenditure will unbalance the diets to the extent that minimal ketosis may occur. It is a good idea to have a small (10 g) portion of readily assimilated carbohydrate available, in case you occasionally feel 'woozy' on these fairly tough, slimming diets. For example, 15 g (½ oz) of biscuits or cookies is a good standby. However, it is always worth remembering that the speed of weight-loss and the efficiency of your diet is indicated by just such 'peculiar' feelings. As these are strict diets for maximum weight-loss you may also feel rather hungry while you are on them.

Obviously the diets can be modified endlessly by consulting the WHAT IS IN FOOD tables in Chapter III. Your health will be safe even if you should decide to stay on the diet for evermore, but, once you get to your average healthy weight, you can increase your total calories, first of all by about 200 calories a day for two or three weeks. If the scales creep up, then cut back again. If weight-loss is maintained, increase your calories to about 1,600 per day, keeping the carbohydrate calories down to 70-80 g (2½-3 oz) of carbohydrate food. Two suitable diets are given in Chapter III.

Counting calories

You do not need a degree in higher mathematics to join the carbohydrate, calorie counters. All you really need is to get to know the equivalent of your bread, fruit and vegetables ingredients. For instance, you can eat about four times the weight of tomatoes as you can peas or potatoes and still consume the same number of calories.

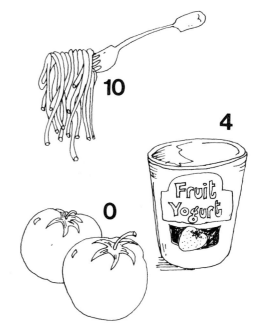

Easy unit dieting

Arithmetic, even the simplest kind, can make some people feel bad. To feel bad when you want to diet makes you feel very bad indeed. To obviate this, Professor John Yudkin devised Unit eating. Based on carbohydrate control, rather than strict calorie counting, it is possible to enjoy a very varied diet but weight-loss is not as certain as it is with the Basic I and II diets.

All foods are divided into three groups and given Unit values. Your daily target is a total of 12 Units.

Group 1 comprises slimmers' free-range foods. They contain no Units and so can be eaten without restriction. This is not the same as saying 'eat as much as you can'. For instance, tomatoes rank as Unit-free in this system, but 100 g (3½ oz) will actually contain 4 g of carbohydrates. If you eat 500 g (1lb 2oz) of tomatoes, you will consume more carbohydrate than you would if you eat a slice of bread. By and large, however, you can gorge on Group 1—and it contains a really fine supply of goodies to make dieting a pleasure.

Group 2 foods should be eaten in moderation, remembering your daily total target is 12 Units taken from Groups 2 and 3.

Group 3 comprises the 'fattening' foods in this dietary regime. While slimming, it is better to get all your Units from Group 2, otherwise they will be used up very quickly, once you spend them in this 'expensive group'.

Group I

No Units - eat as much as you like.

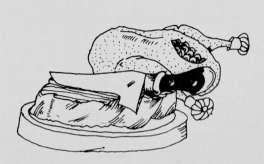
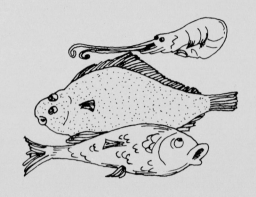

MEAT
Bacon
Beef
Chicken
Duck
Goose
Grouse
Guinea fowl
Ham
Hare
Lamb
Mutton
Partridge
Pheasant.
Pigeon
Pork
Rabbit
Turkey
Veal
Venison

**OFFAL AND
MEAT
PRODUCTS**
Black pudding
Brains
Dripping
Faggots
Heart
Kidneys
Lard
Liver
Liver paste
Liver sausage
Sausage
   (continental)
Suet
Sweetbreads
Tongue
Tripe

FISH
Bloaters
Cockles
Cod
Cod's roe
Crab
Crayfish
Dabs
Dogfish (rock
   salmon)
Eels
Fish paste
Flake
Haddock
Hake
Halibut
Herring
John Dory
Kippers
Ling
Lobster
Mackerel
Mullet

Mussels
Oysters
Pilchards
Plaice
Pollack
Prawns
Salmon
Sardines
Scallops
Shrimps
Skate
Snails
Sole
Sprats
Sturgeon
Trout
Tuna
Turbot
Turtle
Whelks
Whitebait
Whiting
Winkles

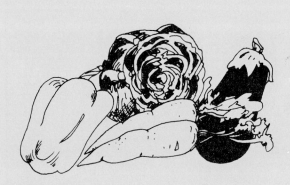

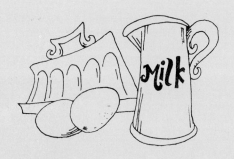

DAIRY PRODUCTS

Butter	Gruyere
Cheese	Parmesan
Camembert	Processed
Cheddar	Roquefort
Cheshire	Stilton
Cottage	Wensleydale
Cream	Cream
Danish blue	Eggs
Edam	Margarine
Emmenthal	Oil
Gorgonzola	cooking
Gouda	salad

GREEN VEGETABLES

Artichoke	Marrow
Asparagus	Mushrooms
Aubergine	Mustard and
Bamboo shoots	cress
Bean sprouts	Olives
Beans	Onions
string	Parsley
runner	Peppers
Broccoli	green
Brussels sprouts	red
Cabbage	Pumpkin
Cauliflower	Radishes
Celery	Rhubarb
Chicory	Sea-kale
Chives	Shallots
Courgettes	Spinach (and
Cucumber	other green
Leeks	leaves)
Lettuce	Spring greens
	Tomatoes
	Watercress

DRINKS

All 'low calorie'	Coffee, black
drinks not	Diet sodas
sweetened	Natural mineral
with sugar or	waters
sorbitol	Soda water
	Tea, black

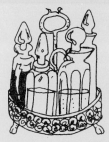

CONDIMENTS AND SAUCES

Bottled sauce	Pepper
Curry powder	Pickles
Ginger	(not sweet)
Gravy	Salad cream
Horseradish	Salt
Mayonnaise	Tomato ketchup
Mustard	Vinegar

Group 2

Because milk is especially rich in nutriments, you
should take at least 275 ml (½ pint) a day.

	Units		Units		Units
Almonds, 30 nuts	½	Gooseberries, fresh 125 g		Pear, fresh 150 g (5 oz)	2½
Apple, fresh 125 g (4 oz)	2	(4 oz)	2	Peas	
Apricot, fresh 125 g (4 oz)	1	Grapefruit (½), fresh	1	dried 25 g (1 oz)	4
Artichoke, Jerusalem 125 g		Grapefruit juice 110 ml		green 125 g (4 oz)	2
(4 oz)	1	(4 fl oz)	2	Pineapple, fresh 125 g	
Avocado (½)	1	Greengages 125 g (4 oz)	2	(4 oz)	2
Beans		Guava 50 g (2 oz)	2	Pineapple juice 110 ml	
baked 125 g (4 oz)	4	Hamburger (1)	1	(4 fl oz)	2½
broad 125 g (4 oz)	3	Hazel nuts, 15 nuts	½	Plums, fresh 125 g (4 oz)	2
butter 125 g (4 oz)	4	Lentils, uncooked 25 g		Pomegranate 50 g (2 oz)	2
haricot 125 g (4 oz)	4	(1 oz)	3	Prunes 25 g (1 oz)	1
kidney 25 g (1 oz)	4	Litchi 50 g (2 oz)	1½	Quince 50 g (2 oz)	2
Beetroot 50 g (2 oz)	1	Loganberries, fresh 125 g		Raisins 25 g (1 oz)	3
Blackberries, fresh 125 g		(4 oz)	1	Raspberries, fresh 125 g	
(4 oz)	2	Mandarins 125 g (4 oz)	2	(4 oz)	2
Brazil nuts, 10 nuts	½	Mango, fresh 125 g (4 oz)	2	Redcurrants, fresh 125 g	
Bread, starch-reduced 25 g		Meat stew 125 g (4 oz)	2	(4 oz)	1
(1 oz)	2	Melon		Roll, starch-reduced,	
Cape gooseberries, fresh		cantaloupe 25 g (1 oz)	1	1 piece	½
125 g (4 oz)	2	honeydew 25 g (1 oz)	2	Sausages (except	
Carrots 75 g (3 oz)	1	water 25 g (1 oz)	1½	continental)	2
Cashew nuts 25 g (1 oz)	1½	Milk, fresh 275 ml		Soups 225 ml (8 fl oz)	2
Cherries, fresh 125 g (4 oz)	3	(½ pint)	3	Soya bean curd 50 g (2 oz)	1
Chestnuts 50 g (2 oz)	4	Mulberries, fresh 125 g		Strawberries, fresh 125 g	
Chickpeas 25 g (1 oz)	4	(4 oz)	2	(4 oz)	1½
Coconut 50 g (2 oz)	3	Nectarines 125 g (4 oz)	2	Sunflower seeds, shelled	1
Crispbread, starch-reduced,		Oranges, fresh 225 g (8 oz)	4	Swede 125 g (4 oz)	1
1 piece	½	Orange juice 110 ml		Sweets 25 g (1 oz)	4
Damsons, fresh 50 g (2 oz)	1	(4 fl oz)	2	Tangerines 125 g (4 oz)	2
Evaporated milk,		Parsnip 125 g (4 oz)	2	Tomato juice 75 ml	
unsweetened 50 ml		Passion fruit 50 g (2 oz)	1	(3 fl oz)	1
(2 fl oz)	1	Pawpaw 175 g (6 oz)	2	Turnip 75 g (3 oz)	1
Fenugreek 25 g (1 oz)	3	Peach, fresh	2	Walnuts, 10 nuts	½
Figs, fresh 125 g (4 oz)	3	Peanuts, 30 nuts	1	Wheat germ 15 g (½ oz)	1
Flour, soya 25 g (1 oz)	1	Peanut butter 25 g (1 oz)	1	Yogurt, plain 150 ml	
				(5 fl oz)	1

Group 3

	Units
Apple dumplings 125 g (4 oz)	4
Apple pie 125 g (4 oz)	7
Apricots in syrup 125 g (4 oz)	5
Arrowroot 25 g (1 oz)	5
Banana 125 g (4 oz)	5
Barley	
uncooked 25 g (1 oz)	4
cooked 75 g (3 oz)	4
Beer and lager 275 ml (½ pint)	5
Biscuits	
sweet, 2 small	3
plain, 3 medium	3
Bitter lemon 225 ml (8 fl oz)	6
Blancmange, 125 g (4 oz)	2
Brandy 25 g (1 fl oz)	4
Bread	
brown 25 g (1 oz)	3
rye 25 g (1 oz)	3
white 25 g (1 oz)	3
Breakfast cereals 25 g (1 oz)	5
starch reduced 25 g (1 oz)	4
Bun	
fruit 50 g (2 oz)	6
iced 50 g (2 oz)	8
plain 50 g (2 oz)	5
Cake	
cream 50 g (2 oz)	7
iced 50 g (2 oz)	8
plain 50 g (2 oz)	7
fruit 50 g (2 oz)	7
Chocolate 50 g (2 oz)	5
Cider 275 ml (½ pint)	7
Condensed milk 50 ml (2 fl oz)	5
Corn (1 cob) 125 g (4 oz)	4
Cornflour 25 g (1 oz)	5
Cottage pie 125 g (4 oz)	3
Cranberry sauce 25 g (1 oz)	2½
Crispbread (not starch reduced), 1 piece	2½
Custard	
egg 125 g (4 oz)	2
powder 125 g (4 oz)	2
Dates, dried 25 g (1 oz)	4
Doughnut 50 g (2 oz)	6
Figs	
dried 25 g (1 oz)	3

	Units
in syrup 125 g (4 oz)	8
Flour 25 g (1 oz)	4
Fructose 15 g (½ oz)	3
Fruit juice, canned, sweetened 110 ml (4 fl oz)	3
Gin 25 ml (1 fl oz)	4
Ginger ale 225 ml (8 fl oz)	6
dry 225 ml (8 fl oz)	4
Ginger beer 225 ml (8 fl oz)	6
Glucose 50 g (2 oz)	3
Glucose drink 175 ml (6 fl oz)	6
Golden syrup 25 g (1 oz)	4
Gooseberries in syrup 125 g (4 oz)	5
Grapefruit juice, sweetened 50 ml (2 fl oz)	3
Grapes 125 g (4 oz)	3
Honey 25 g (1 oz)	5
Ice-cream 50 g (2 oz)	3
Jam 15 g (½ oz)	2
Jelly 125 g (4 oz)	4
Lemonade 225 ml (8 fl oz)	5
Lemon curd 15 g (½ oz)	2
Liqueurs 25 ml (1 fl oz)	5
Macaroni	
cheese 125 g (4 oz)	5
plain, cooked 175 g (6 oz)	10
Maize 25 g (1 oz)	4
Mandarins in syrup 125 g (4 oz)	4
Marmalade 15 g (½ oz)	2
Milk pudding 125 g (4 oz)	5
Millet 25 g (1 oz)	4
Mince pies 50 g (2 oz)	5
Noodles, cooked	9
Oatcake 25 g (1 oz)	3
Oatmeal	
uncooked 25 g (1 oz)	3
cooked 175 g (6 oz)	3
Orange juice, sweetened 110 ml (4 fl oz)	3
Pancakes 50 g (2 oz)	4
Pastry 25 g (1 oz)	3
Peaches in syrup 125 g (4 oz)	5
Pears in syrup 125 g (4 oz)	5
Pineapple in syrup 125 g (4 oz)	5
Plantain 125 g (4 oz)	7
Plums in syrup 125 g (4 oz)	5

	Units
Plum pudding 75 g (3 oz)	9
Pork pie 125 g (4 oz)	4
Port 50 ml (2 fl oz)	4
Potato 75 g (3 oz)	3
crisps 25 g (1 oz)	3
Raspberries in syrup 125 g (4 oz)	5
Rhubarb pie 125 g (4 oz)	6
Rice, cooked 125 g (4 oz)	5
Roll 50 g (2 oz)	6
Sago pudding 125 g (4 oz)	4
Scone 50 g (2 oz)	6
Semolina pudding 125 g (4 oz)	4
Sherry 50 ml (2 fl oz)	4
Sorbitol 15 g (½ oz)	3
Spaghetti, cooked 175 g (6 oz)	10
Steak and kidney pie 125 g (4 oz)	4
pudding 125 g (4 oz)	4
Stout 275 ml (½ pint)	6
Strawberries in syrup 125 g (4 oz)	5
Sugar	
brown 15 g (½ oz)	3
white 15 g (½ oz)	3
Sweet potatoes 75 g (3 oz)	5
Sweets, boiled 25 g (1 oz)	4
Syrup 15 g (½ oz)	2½
Tangerines in syrup 125 g (4 oz)	5
Tapioca	
cooked 125 g (4 oz)	4
pudding 125 g (4 oz)	5
Toffees 25 g (1 oz)	4
Tonic water 175 ml (6 fl oz)	2½
Treacle 15 g (½ oz)	2½
Vermicelli, cooked 175 g (6 oz)	9
Vermouth	
sweet 50 ml (2 fl oz)	5
dry 50 ml (2 fl oz)	3
Whisky 25 ml (1 fl oz)	4
Wine	
dry 75 ml (3 fl oz)	3
sweet 75 ml (3 fl oz)	4
Yogurt, flavoured 150 ml (5 fl oz)	4
Yorkshire pudding 50 g (2 oz)	5

A week of Unit dieting

Using the Unit principle, it is possible to work out a tremendously varied diet. Here is an example of a week's meals following the Unit dieting system.

	MONDAY (In addition you may use a further 3 units from the guide.)	TUESDAY (In addition you may use a further 1½ units from the guide.)	WEDNESDAY (In addition you may use a further 1½ units from the guide.)
	Units	Units	Units
BREAKFAST	½ glass grapefruit juice, unsweetened 1 Fried egg and bacon 0 Tea or coffee with milk, no sugar 1 1 starch-reduced crispbread ½ Butter 0	Orange juice, unsweetened 2 Boiled egg 0 ½ slice bread 1½ Butter 0 Tea or coffee with milk, no sugar 1	Fried kipper 0 ½ slice bread 1½ Butter 0 Tea or coffee with milk, no sugar 1
LUNCH	Cheese or mushroom omelet (2 eggs) 0 2 starch-reduced crispbreads 1 Butter 0 Tea or coffee with milk, no sugar 1	Cheese 0 Green salad 0 Tomato 0 1 starch-reduced crispbread ½ Butter 0 Tea or coffee with milk, no sugar 1	2 grilled or fried sausages 2 1 grilled tomato 0 2 starch-reduced crispbreads 1 Butter 0 Cheese 0 Tea or coffee with milk, no sugar 1
DINNER	Braised liver including carrots, onions, turnip, celery 1½ Fresh fruit salad, cream 2 Tea or coffee with milk, no sugar 1	Mushroom soup 2 Grilled or fried cod fillets, parsley 0 50 g (2 oz) peas 1 1 starch-reduced crispbread ½ Butter, cheese 0 Tea or coffee with milk, no sugar 1	Consomme 0 Roast chicken 0 Brussels sprouts 0 Stewed rhubarb, saccharine to sweeten 0 Tea or coffee with milk, no sugar 1 1 glass dry white wine 3
	TOTAL 9	**TOTAL** 10½	**TOTAL** 10½

THURSDAY	FRIDAY	SATURDAY	SUNDAY
(In addition you may use a further 1½ units from the guide.)	(In addition you may use a further 4 units from the guide.)	(In addition you may use a further 3½ units from the guide.)	(In addition you may use a further 2½ units from the guide.)
Units	**Units**	**Units**	**Units**
Poached egg — 0	½ grapefruit — 1	½ grapefruit — 1	Smoked haddock — 0
½ slice toast — 1½	Grilled or fried bacon — 0	Fried egg and bacon — 0	1 starch-reduced
Butter — 0	Grilled or fried	½ slice bread — 1½	crispbread — ½
Tea or coffee with milk,	mushrooms — 0	Butter — 0	Butter — 0
no sugar — 1	Tea or coffee with milk,	Tea or coffee with milk,	Tea or coffee with milk,
	no sugar — 1	no sugar — 1	no sugar — 1
Fried fish — 0	Ham — 0	Stewed beef — 0	Roast beef — 0
50 g (2 oz) peas — 1	Tomato, lettuce,	Brussels sprouts — 0	1 medium potato — 3
2 starch-reduced	cucumber, radishes — 0	Fresh fruit salad — 2	Cabbage — 0
crispbreads — 1	Apple — 2	Cream — 0	2 starch-reduced
Butter — 0	150 ml (5 fl oz) milk — 1½	Tea or coffee with milk,	crispbreads — 1
Cheese — 0		no sugar — 1	Butter, cheese — 0
Tea or coffee with milk,			Tea or coffee with milk,
no sugar — 1			no sugar — 1
Mushroom soup — 2	Consomme — 0	Grilled or fried fish — 0	Consomme — 0
Lamb chops — 0	Stewed beef — 0	Spinach — 0	Ham — 0
Cabbage — 0	Carrots — 1	2 starch-reduced	Green salad — 0
Fresh fruit salad — 2	1 starch-reduced	crispbreads — 1	Fresh fruit salad — 2
Cream — 0	crispbread — ½	Butter — 0	Cream — 0
Tea or coffee with milk,	Butter and cheese — 0	Cheese — 0	Tea or coffee with milk,
no sugar — 1	Tea or coffee with milk,	Tea or coffee with milk,	no sugar — 1
	no sugar — 1	no sugar — 1	
TOTAL — 10½	**TOTAL — 8**	**TOTAL — 8½**	**TOTAL — 9½**

CHAPTER V

The high fat diet

High fat diets are extremely effective and are based on sound scientific principles, backed by modern research.

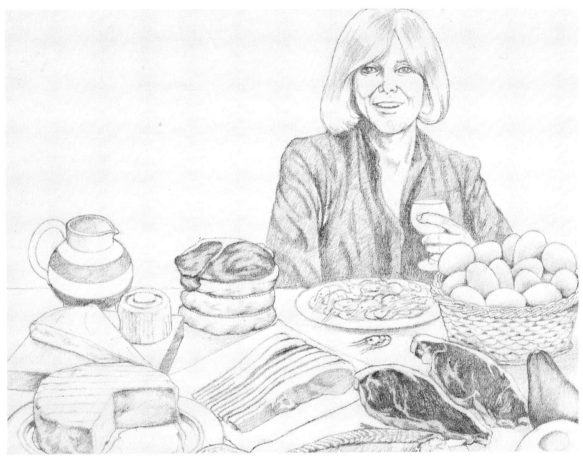

It is a pity that high fat diets are a bit out of fashion at the moment. Perhaps they sound unappetizing, but fashions change. As it happens, they are really quite exciting and extremely effective. One very important bonus of a high fat diet is that it has in-built staying power. In other words, when you are on a high fat slimming diet, it is very unusual to feel hungry, weak or liable to raid the refrigerator, or to develop into a secret eater and thus ruin your chances of weight reduction. The people who should think twice before embarking on a high fat diet are the elderly, who may find it difficult to digest large quantities of fat.

How it works

Punters in the slimming field invariably 'go off' fats when they study their calorie charts. This is understandable, for, weight for weight, fat is absolutely packed with calories. Then how can you lose weight by eating foods very high in calories? The answer, like the answer to any

nutrition question, is not completely understood. Nevertheless, it is a fact that you can eat a high fat diet of 2,000-3,000 calories per day and still lose 3-5 kg (7-12 lb) a month. In other words, you can diet without ever feeling hungry and to do so, you only have to follow two quite basic rules.

1 **Virtually eliminate carbohydrate from your diet.**
2 **Live on fat and protein foods in the proportion of one part of fat to three parts of protein.**

The most likely reason for the success of high fat diets is that they stoke up the body's internal fires and stimulate the production of more energy, as heat and internal chemical reactions. People on high fat diets tend to feel nicely warm, not hot, themselves and warm to the touch of others. In a way they have got their body energy processes—their internal fires—set at 'high'. But this is only a partial explanation of what is happening to them and it is quite difficult to understand the whole picture. This is because we all tend to turn to mechanical models or systems, like stoking engines, to try to understand how body processes work. These can help but no machine works exactly like the human body. For example, those who have tried to 'explain' why high fat diets are so effective have talked about fat being like the bellows kindling up a fire, or working like the damper or draught regulator on a boiler. Of course, in industrial terms, if you want a lot of energy, in the form of heat, to produce steam and drive a turbine which, in turn, produces the electricity that powers a factory, all you have to do to the boiler is to open the damper and let in more air. The increased airflow makes the fire burn faster.

As far as it goes, this is a reasonable analogy for high fat slimming, but it is somewhat unrealistic. Our body temperature, for example, stays roughly the same all the time, whatever we eat. We have no 'fires' burning in our bodies in the conventional sense. However, every tiny cell in the body is a complex, molecular powerhouse, a miniature factory for making everything the body requires. Our cellular tissues also break down the things that we do not need and which, if they were allowed to accumulate, would poison us. All of these body processes need energy to function. That energy comes ultimately from the food we eat or from stored fat.

The type of energy with which we provide our cells influences the rate at which it is consumed. In the same way that a peat fire burns slowly and dry firewood burns up brightly and quickly, the fat or carbohydrate that we supply to our cells will alter the character of our internal 'fires'. Nutritional scientists would say that our rate of metabolism is altered.

One way of looking at this idea is to consider a pile of compost rotting away at the bottom of your garden. The compost heap has, of course, a function. It is to produce simple substances which later on can be mixed into the soil to feed next season's plants. The various vegetables and flowers that stock our summer gardens depend on 'processed' compost. Compost heaps rot-down or are processed quickly or slowly depending on their composition. If you mix plenty of lawn cuttings into the heap, the compost 'works' fast. This is because all the complicated chemical reactions going on invisibly inside it are proceeding at high speed. Often the chemical turnover is so fast you can feel it on the surface as heat. So the grass cuttings 'work', in their vegetable way, a bit like fat does in an animal system. Whether or not your compost heap shrinks down and is ready to use on the garden in three months or in two years

depends on its finely-chopped, green contents. In a similar way, the amount of fat (grass) that we feed to our bodies (compost heaps) decides whether we stay fat or grow slim.

Unlike the compost heap, we do not actually get hotter as we use up our stores of energy. This is largely because our body compensates for this by losing more heat. This prevents our temperature rising and gives a clue to the slimming nature of fat. On a high fat diet, 30-50 per cent of the weight lost by the slimmer leaves as water. Mostly this is lost through what scientists call insensible, or dry, perspiration. It evaporates from our skin before it forms into beads of sweat and so we do not notice it. The rest of the weight-loss results from using the stored body fat for the metabolic processes, giving us the energy we need to live and move about.

Scientific research

Some slimmers like to know a bit more about how their diets affect their bodies and to learn something of the scientific background to their particular diets. The high fat diet is based on sound scientific principles and is backed by modern research.

Results of recent animal and human studies have shown that body weight is not directly related to calorie intake. Instead, researchers suggest that much obesity results from the inability of certain people to 'burn off' excess calories they have eaten, as heat. These excess calories are then stored as fat.

New theories have shown, however, that not all body fat is the same. There are two kinds of body fat—simple storage fat and brown fat. Brown fat is closely involved with the production of heat within the body. Dr Michael Stock of Queen Elizabeth College, London, and American and Canadian research groups, led by Dr George A. Bray of the Division of Metabolism and Nutrition, University of California, have shown that overfeeding normal animals increases body heat production in rats and humans, and that this process occurs in the body's brown fat. Rats kept in laboratories are fussy eaters and usually eat just enough to keep their body weights constant. Researchers designed diets heavily laced with chocolate, sausages and fat that tempted rats to eat more. In one experiment the rats consumed 80 per cent more calories and gained 27 per cent more weight. Their metabolic rates, which are an indication of general cell activity, also increased considerably on this regime. So too did the amount of brown fat they had in their bodies. In fact, in three weeks, they had doubled the amount of brown fat in their bodies. Once the rats were taken off their fattening diets, they quickly lost weight because their brown fat was rapidly burning up energy.

Experimental research has shown areas in the human body where similar brown fat tends to lie. It is deposited in the neck and the upper back particularly. Drugs, such as ephedrene, can be used to give an artificial stimulus to the body's general metabolic process, for a short time. When ephedrene was given to human volunteers, special heat measurements, called thermograms, showed which areas of the body had become metabolically active, that is, which areas were producing a lot of heat. It has been shown that these areas are the places where most brown fat is normally deposited. These experiments confirm the clinical impressions and the reasoned arguments of Dr Richard Mackarness, who first advocated and popularized high fat diets as aids to slimming in his book, *Eat Fat and Grow Slim*, published in 1958.

High fat diets work for two fundamental reasons. They allow people to alter their bad eating habits by providing an energy-rich diet, which they can maintain and which is not, if properly balanced, productive of fat on the body. This diet, probably by increasing the body's brown fat store, burns off storage fat as heat and water. Moreover, once formed, the brown fat, with its high metabolic activity, seems to 'remain' in the body to cope with extra calories and maintain the slimming diet. A high fat diet is the only one that seems to 'keep on working', for some people at least, so that they do not put on weight once they go back to ordinary eating habits.

Getting down to it

The actual food you eat on a high fat diet can vary considerably. However, the diet must be based on the following 'do's and don'ts' to make it work.

DO
1 **Eat as much of your diet as you want to keep feeling full and satisfied.**
2 **There must be one part of fat to three parts of protein (by weight) in all the food you eat.**
3 **Drink plenty—at least 1.7 litres (3 pints) of liquid per day (for example water, unsweetened coffee with milk or cream, unsweetened black**

coffee, unsweetened tea without milk, unsweetened fruit juice.)
4 **Take as much seasoning and dressing as you like, except salt.**

DON'T
1 **Eat carbohydrate or sugary foods (except when matched by fat/protein equivalents—see below).**
2 **Take added salt with meals.**

Sample menus

A little later we will go into the ways and means of making a high fat diet pleasantly varied and, sometimes, positively scrumptious. To start with, we give a sample week's menus.

A quick appraisal shows the areas where you have to change your eating patterns. In other words no milk, sugar, confectionery, bread, flour or thickening are permitted. Artificial sweeteners are allowed. Tea certainly becomes a strange meal and the lack of bread, crispbread and toast takes a bit of getting used to. Nevertheless, it is worth persevering because this diet works and keeps you fit and losing weight without feeling deprived.

Slimmer's gourmet guide

If you have not got much time to work out diets and meals, the advice detailed above will get you slim. But it is possible to be very much more adventurous by designing your own high fat diet, using the following system (see page 62).

Meat, fish and poultry 'staple foods' are graded 1st, 2nd and 3rd class, according to their fat content. These can all be eaten with impunity. Where no class is given, the food is low on fat and must be balanced, weight for weight, with a 1st class food or a double-sized portion of a 2nd class food. 3rd class foods contain equal parts of fat and protein. Zero-rated items are suspect, as they contain more protein than fat.

Vegetables and fruit are classed under three headings. **F** means they contain so little carbohydrate that they can be freely taken. **M** means matched vegetables and these must always be matched with the equal parts of a 1st class food, or a double quantity of a 2nd class food. **O** foods contain medium quantities of carbohydrates and can be matched with an equal quantity of 3rd class foods, or half as much 1st or 2nd class foods. **X** rated foods contain enough carbohydrate to spoil your slimming chances. Alcohol, in the form of dry white wine and spirits, is allowed in only moderate amounts.

A week at a glance

All the items are interchangeable. If cost is a problem, pick out the less expensive ones and substitute others. Lunch and dinner are interchangeable.

Remember
1 **No sugar, no bread or flour for thickening.**
2 **No added salt. Synthetics may be used for sweetening.**
3 **There is no restriction on water. Drink at least 1.7 litres (3 pints) a day, flavoured with fresh lemon juice if you like it.**
4 **Non-fish-eaters should take a tablespoonful of cod-liver oil daily or eat two capsules of cod-liver oil with each meal.**

	MONDAY	TUESDAY	WEDNESDAY	
BREAKFAST	Unsweetened fruit juice Haddock (large portion) stewed in milk with 2 pats of butter Coffee with cream or top of milk Starch-reduced rolls with plenty of butter	Half grapefruit (no sweetening) 2 slices bacon and fried egg Coffee with cream or top of milk Starch-reduced roll with plenty of butter or margarine	Half grapefruit (no sweetening) Kippers or herrings Fried tomatoes Coffee and cream or top of milk	
LUNCH	Half grapefruit (no sweetening) Sardines, and salad Fresh fruit salad (unsweetened) and fresh cream Coffee and cream	Sliced cucumber and dressing Fried veal steak with gravy French beans or cauliflower Cheese souffle or Cheddar cheese	Tomato juice Soused herrings Peas Brie or Cheddar cheese	
TEA	Lemon tea Slice of cheese	Lemon tea Plain yogurt	Lemon tea Fresh fruit and cream	
DINNER	Beef steak Fried tomatoes or mushrooms Salad Celery	Clear vegetable soup Canned salmon or tuna Green salad and tomatoes, with oil and vinegar dressing Cream cheese Coffee black (or with cream)	Asparagus soup (no thickening) Lamb, mint sauce Broad beans with butter, spinach (average portion) Plums (unsweetened) and cream	

THURSDAY	FRIDAY	SATURDAY	SUNDAY
Fresh orange Fresh ham with fat Fried egg Coffee with cream or top of milk Starch-reduced rolls	Fresh fruit Canned fish Tomato Coffee and cream	Half grapefruit (no sweetening) Omelet Coffee and cream or top of milk Starch-reduced rolls with plenty of butter	Fruit juice (no sweetening) Eggs, scrambled with butter Coffee and cream or top of milk 2 starch-reduced rolls with butter or margarine and yeast extract
Cold buttered prawns or canned herring or pilchard Green salad with mayonnaise Gruyere cheese Coffee and cream	Grapefruit Steak and salad with French dressing Cheese Coffee and cream	Slices of melon Canned fish Salad with mixed dressing Rhubarb (unsweetened) with cream	Roast beef Chips (small portion) or baked potato, marrow or courgettes Fresh fruit salad (unsweetened) and cream Coffee with cream
Lemon tea Celery	Lemon tea Yogurt	Lemon tea Slice of cheese	
Fruit juice Large portion of beef stew with mixed vegetables (no potatoes) and mushrooms Coffee with cream	Offal with onions, Brussels sprouts or cabbage Cheese Large coffee and cream	Avocado pear and salad dressing Liver and bacon fried with large portion creamed spinach and mushrooms Coffee and cream	Canned fish and salad or coleslaw Fresh pineapple with cream Black coffee

Gourmet guide
MEAT, POULTRY AND GAME

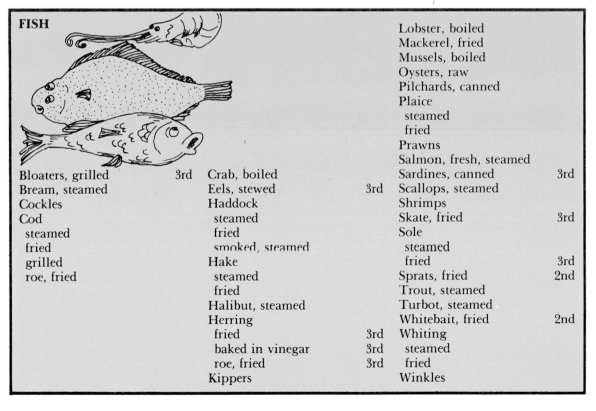

				Kidney		
				stewed		
				fried		
				Lamb		
				chop, grilled, lean		
				and fat	1st	
				leg, roast	3rd	
				scrag and neck, stewed	3rd	
Bacon				Liver, fried		
average	2nd			Pheasant, roast		
fore end	2nd	Brains, boiled		Pork		
middle	2nd	Chicken		leg, roast	3rd	
gammon	2nd	boiled		loin, roast, lean and fat		
Beef		roast		chops, grilled	1st	
corned		Dripping, beef	1st	Rabbit, stewed		
silverside, boiled	3rd	Duck, roast		Tongue	2nd	
sirloin, lean and fat	2nd	Goose, roast		Tripe, stewed		
steak, fried	3rd	Grouse, roast		Turkey, roast		
steak, grilled	3rd	Ham, boiled, lean and fat	2nd	Veal cutlet, fried		
stewed		Heart, roast		Venison, roast		

FISH

				Lobster, boiled	
				Mackerel, fried	
				Mussels, boiled	
				Oysters, raw	
				Pilchards, canned	
				Plaice	
				steamed	
				fried	
				Prawns	
				Salmon, fresh, steamed	
Bloaters, grilled	3rd	Crab, boiled		Sardines, canned	3rd
Bream, steamed		Eels, stewed	3rd	Scallops, steamed	
Cockles		Haddock		Shrimps	
Cod		steamed		Skate, fried	3rd
steamed		fried		Sole	
fried		smoked, steamed		steamed	
grilled		Hake		fried	3rd
roe, fried		steamed		Sprats, fried	2nd
		fried		Trout, steamed	
		Halibut, steamed		Turbot, steamed	
		Herring		Whitebait, fried	2nd
		fried	3rd	Whiting	
		baked in vinegar	3rd	steamed	
		roe, fried	3rd	fried	
		Kippers		Winkles	

VEGETABLES

Asparagus	F
Beans	
broad, boiled	O
French	F
haricot	X
runner	F
Beetroot	X
Brussels sprouts	F
Cabbage	F
Carrots	O
Cauliflower	F
Celery	
raw	F
boiled	F
Chicory	F
Cucumber	F
Leeks	M
Lettuce	F
Marrow	F
Mushrooms	F
Onions	F
Parsnips	X
Peas	O
Potatoes, boiled	X
Radishes	F
Spinach	F
Spring greens	F
Swedes	O
Tomatoes, raw	F
Turnips	F
Watercress	F

FRUITS

Stewed fruit must not be sweetened with sugar. Canned fruit should be avoided.

Apples		Grapes	
dessert	O	black	O
baked	O	white	O
stewed	O	Grapefruit	F
Apricots		Greengages, stewed	O
fresh	O	Lemon juice	F
dried and stewed	X	Loganberries	F
Bananas	X	Melons, cantaloupe	O
Blackberries		Oranges	O
fresh	O	Orange juice	O
stewed	O	Peaches	O
Cherries	O	Pears	
Damsons		fresh	O
fresh	O	stewed	O
stewed	O	Pineapple	O
Figs	O	Plums	
Gooseberries, stewed	F	fresh	O
		stewed	O
		Prunes, stewed	O
		Raspberries, stewed	O
		Rhubarb, stewed	F
		Strawberries	O

NUTS

Almonds	O	Coconut	
Barcelona	O	fresh	O
Brazil	O	desiccated	O
Chestnuts	X	Peanuts	O
Cob nuts	O	Walnuts	O
		Olives (with stone)	F

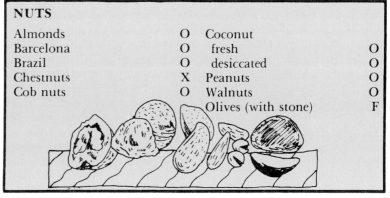

Key

Meat, fish and staple foods

1st class foods	Eat as much as you like
2nd class foods	Eat as much as you like
3rd class foods (contain equal parts of fat and protein)	Eat as much as you like
Zero rated foods (contain more protein than fat)	Avoid if possible

Vegetables and fruit

F (contain very little carbohydrate)	Eat as much as you like
M (matched vegetables)	Match with equal parts of a 1st class food or a double quantity of a 2nd class food
O (contain medium quantities of carbohydrates)	Match with an equal quantity of a 3rd class food or half as much of a 1st or 2nd class food
X (high in carbohydrates)	Avoid
Alcohol	Small quantities of dry white wine and spirits allowed

Speeding up the weight-loss

With the standard diet regime, Mr and Mrs Average lose about 1.5-3 kg (3-7 lb) a week. To increase the rate of weight-loss, pep up your body processes more by adding the following boost factors into your high fat slimming routine.

1 **Set your alarm clock earlier, so that you always sleep less than seven hours per night (weight-loss is quicker awake than asleep).**
2 **Drink a 275 ml (½ pint) of water and then walk briskly for half an hour per day before breakfast. (This is in addition and not an alternative to your everyday normal exercise.) It puts your body into gear for using up fat before the day really starts and you tend to stay at this metabolic rate all day.**
3 **Drink 575 ml (1 pint) of water or fruit juice between breakfast and lunch.**
4 **Take a token walk after lunch and dinner. Ten minutes will do.**
5 **Abolish all alcoholic drinks from your routine.**

Facts and fallacies

No diet is perfect, but there are many ways of sabotaging all diets. The sabotage can be self-inflicted, to avoid having to follow the diet, or caused by well-meaning friends or neighbours, who feel you are damaging your health. Knowing the objections and the fallacies helps you keep to the diet and lose weight.

Heart disease

Fallacy 1 If you eat too much fat you will get heart disease (coronary disease) and suffer from high blood pressure.

The Facts We do not know all the facts about heart disease and its relationship to what we eat. We do know that the fat content of the blood is very variable and related both to the type of fat eaten and to stress and exercise. We also know that overfat people suffer far more from heart disease and stroke than thinner people. The oils and fats we eat are essential to control the blood's clotting mechanism and, if this is defective, we are at hazard if we are injured or have surgery. It seems likely that two opposite, fatty factors are operating in the blood. The fats in the foods we eat produce in the body two naturally opposing substances—prostacyclins and thromboxane. Prostacyclins tend to open up blood vessels and prevent clot formation. Thromboxane closes blood vessels and promotes clotting. Animal and vegetable fats tend to make more thromboxane than prostacyclin. Fish fats tip the balance in favour of prostacyclin.

In countries where the usual diet contains a high proportion of fish fat, relatively few people die as a result of thrombosis-type diseases. (They also tend to bleed heavily after having a tooth out, particularly Eskimos, whose main source of fat is from fish.) In places where animal fat predominates in the diet, the reverse is true. Our menus cleverly match fish and animal fat to give a safe balance. People who dislike fish should take cod-liver oil in the form of oil made into salad dressing or as capsules taken with meals.

Gall bladder disease

Fallacy 2 High fat diets are sickly and give you gall bladder disease (gallstones).

The Facts If you already have gall bladder disease, you will have trouble digesting fat, and another type of diet will probably be best for you. However, there is no evidence that high fat intake predisposes to gall bladder or any other disease, if the fat eaten is matched well (see above).

The complaint that fat is sickly is purely a culinary matter. People who traditionally eat high fat diets know the value of herbs, condiments, fruit juices and vinegars, which, if skilfully used, make fat delicious to eat. In fact, your diet always contains more fat than you think. Meat, usually thought of as 'pure' protein, actually contains about 50 per cent fat, even if you remove most of it before cooking.

Ketosis

Fallacy 3 If you suddenly stop eating carbohydrates (bread, sugar, flour products etc) and eat a lot of fat, you have to go through a period of ketosis, when you feel strange and may become ill or develop diabetes.

The Facts Nobody becomes ill on a high fat diet. Ketosis is an accumulation in the body of substances, which are related to acetone, and their subsequent appearance in the urine and in the breath, where they smell sweet and aromatic. They are evidence that the body is burning up a lot of fat in the absence of carbohydrate as 'fuel'. A degree of ketosis is produced by all effective diets because the body is using its store of fat for 'fuel'. More information about ketosis is given in Chapter I.

Sometimes mood changes are associated with the mild ketosis of weight reduction. Some people become a bit irritable and bad-tempered and others become slightly 'high', as though they have had a couple of alcoholic drinks.

The confusion about the unhealthiness of ketosis probably stems from the fact that diabetics, whose disease is not under proper control, often suffer from severe ketosis. Because diabetes prevents the body from dealing with carbohydrates, it attempts to burn up masses of body fat at a very high rate. This produces a lot of ketones, perhaps 30 times more than results from the high fat diet recommended for slimmers.

Unnatural or harmful

Fallacy 4 High fat diets are unnatural and, therefore, harmful.

The Facts Leaving aside the fact that primitive Man probably lived on a high fat diet before he eventually took to agriculture, there is no evidence of an 'unnatural' or 'harmful' factor operating in the high fat diet described. Some people still live permanently on high fat diets, notably the Eskimo in his natural way of life.

Eskimos remain slim while on this diet, but rapidly fatten up on Western diets.

Summer dieting

Fallacy 5 High fat diets are too 'hot' for dieting in the summer.

The Facts The body deals with all internally generated heat in the same way. The majority of body cooling is brought about by insensible, or unfelt, perspiration, whereby sweat evaporates from the skin surface as quickly as it is secreted. People on high fat diets feel warm to touch, but do not experience any sensation of being hotter than anybody else.

Diet fibre

Fallacy 6 High fat diets make you constipated because they contain no fibre from bread.

The Facts The diet provides a generous allowance of salads and unlimited green beans, Brussels sprouts, cauliflower, celery, chicory, cucumber, lettuce, marrow, mushrooms, onions, radishes, spinach, spring greens, tomatoes, turnips and watercress, all of which keep the bowels regular. Fibre, in the form of bran, can be added to the diet for those with sluggish bowels.

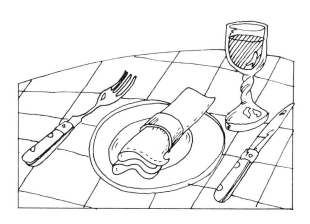

CHAPTER VI

The high protein diet

Protein forms an essential part of Man's diet. High protein diets require no calorie counting and result in rapid initial weight-loss. They are especially suitable for children and adolescents who need plenty of body-building protein in their diet.

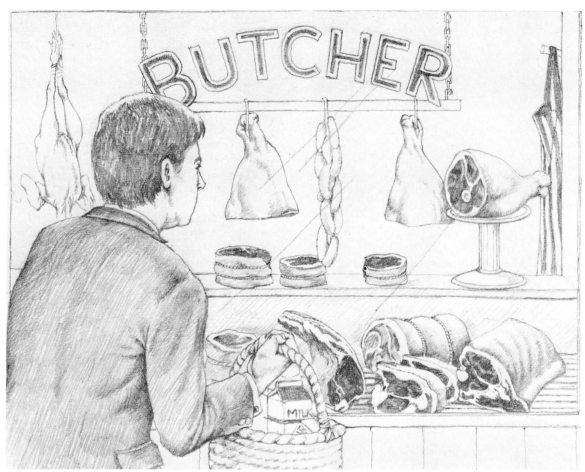

Protein plays a special role in keeping the body healthy. It is possible to maintain a healthy equilibrium without two of the three important building bricks that make up the food we eat—carbohydrate and fat. However, if we try to live on a diet totally deficient in protein, we soon become ill and eventually die. Indeed, the signs and symptoms of starvation are those of lack of protein. Strangely, we can survive on protein alone, for the body has the capacity to use protein for the maintenance of health or to burn it to produce vital energy.

Why is protein special?

Protein's unique place in health results from two biological facts of life. First, we cannot make protein from carbohydrate and fat, the other main components of the food we eat. Second, every one of us, as we sit reading this book, lying in bed or running for the bus, is using up, or, in effect, losing protein.

This protein drain is partly due to growth and adequate protein in all diets for growing children and young people is, therefore, vital. It is important to realize, however, that even adults are still 'growing'. Obviously, if we suddenly decide to take more regular exercise we 'grow' more muscle, but we also 'grow' all the time in other ways. Our skin is continually flaking off and being replaced. So too are all the mucous membranes, the tissues which line the mouth, stomach, digestive tract, bowels, bladder and vagina. In addition, these tissues produce lubricating mucus, which is also a protein substance. We grow in other ways and so lose protein, such as in our hair and nails. Supplies of vital protein are necessary for the constant renewal of blood (red blood cells, especially, have a very short effective life and have to be replaced constantly). Hormones, such as the sex and thyroid hormones, needed to keep vital processes ticking over, as well as the enzymes necessary to digest the food we eat, are protein substances.

What all this really amounts to is that a regular intake of protein is absolutely and literally vital to Man's survival. The amount of protein required is not actually very much—about 70 g (2½ oz) a day is plenty—but without it, we would die.

Vital proteins

Naturally enough, all diets, even vegetarian diets, need to be planned around this nutritional kernel of protein. Moreover, plenty of protein has for dieters, quite rightly, a ring of reassuring authenticity about it. There is another factor about protein of interest to slimmers. Our bodies, especially bodies similar to that of Mr Constant Weight, do not store all the excess food we eat. If we eat more food and, therefore, more calories than we need to balance our output of energy, the body promptly 'steps up' its energy output to a higher level, behaving (happily, the slimmer will say) in a rather spendthrift manner. Protein tends to turn the occasional spendthrift into a veritable rake, as far as energy output is concerned. The intake of any food switches the level of fuel expenditure up by about five per cent. But protein foods really burn up the wick of nutrition to the extent of 30-37 per cent.

The protein bonus

This curious characteristic of protein, so helpful to the dieter, is called its specific dynamic action. When scientists invent a rather splendid and impressive name for a biological process, it is a sure sign that they do not know very much about it. In fact, the whole principle of specific dynamic action is obscure.

Nevertheless, we do know something about it. We know that there is little specific dynamic action (or prodigal calorie loss), when we are out and about in cold weather. Perhaps this is because the body uses extra protein as simple fuel. There is also little specific dynamic action when protein is needed in large quantities for body repair work, such as after blood loss or severe burning. In such cases, we need all the protein we can assimilate for repair processes. These two facts are of minimal concern to slimmers, but the third known fact about specific dynamic action is really very interesting and is the main reason for thinking about high protein dieting. Specific dynamic action appears to be most effective when more protein is eaten than is necessary to replace wear and tear. In other words, the more protein you eat,

the more you 'waste', from the point of view of nutrition. This 'throw-away' effect, as far as calories are concerned, can be of great advantage to the slimmer.

High protein diets have one big disadvantage—high protein foods tend to be expensive. Therefore, high protein diets are not feasible to those who have to balance food expenditure in terms of money as well as in terms of weight-loss.

High protein diets do not seem to have any medical disadvantages, despite the fact that all the protein we eat in excess of the body's needs for replacement and wear and tear, is apparently 'tossed on to the bonfires of the body, there to provide an extravagant and useless waste of heat, not only by the combustion of its component amino acids (the building bricks of proteins) but of fat and carbohydrates as well'—as one prominent, nutritional scientist put it. The Eskimo, whose life is much closer to nature than our own, eats five times as much protein as we do, but has no greater health problems and does not suffer from obesity.

Two ways to diet

From the practical point of view, high protein diets fall into two categories—those which produce ketosis and those which do not. Ketosis is a condition which occurs because there is an acute lack of carbohydrate in the diet (see Chapter I). High protein diets which do not produce ketosis restrict the amount of carbohydrate consumed, while allowing the dieter to continue to eat as much protein as before. The ketosis-producing, high protein diets contain almost no carbohydrate and give added protein. Some of these diets utilize the subsequent ketosis to monitor their progress (see Chapter VIII).

The built-in joy of high protein

High protein diets have several hidden bonuses for those who want to lose weight. Unlike calorie reduction diets, high protein diets produce a rapid initial weight-loss. Much of this is due to water loss, so there is a tendency for the scales to 'stick' for a while later. Even so, weight-loss is maintained and, provided slimmers know about it, they usually accept it cheerfully.

Another advantage of high protein diets is that they are very suitable for children. They also appeal to those who feel that food is intrinsically good for them and that food deprivation is bad.

High protein diets are very useful to overweight people who, for business reasons, eat regularly in restaurants. It is very easy to find high protein food in restaurants at the *haute cuisine* end of the scale, although rather more difficult, but not impossible, to find it in most modest diners. Nevertheless, eggs and basic meat dishes are usually available to those for whom eating away from home is a part of everyday living. Salads and low carbohydrate vegetables from the WHAT IS IN FOOD list in Chapter III can be chosen. Finally, high protein diets can offer to the slimmer the promise he most desperately wants to hear—he need never feel hungry.

High protein dieting

On a high protein diet you do not have to count the calories. High protein foods are meat, poultry, fish and eggs and you may also eat foods from the permitted list given below. On no account should you stray into the non-permitted category. You may eat as much as you need to stop feeling hungry but, clearly, you must be sensible about the size of your main high protein portions. If you eat a leg of lamb or a whole chicken every day you are going to fail on this sort of diet. Frequent small meals are preferable to large ones.

General rules

1 Do not count calories.
2 Eat the permitted foods to avoid hunger, but do not eat when you are not hungry.
3 Do not feel that you must finish everything on your plate.
4 Frequent small meals are preferable to large ones.
5 Drink as much water or calorie-free drinks with no carbohydrate content as you like. Do not restrict fluids, but do not force them either.
6 Do not drink milk or alcohol.
7 Take a multivitamin pill daily.
8 Do not eat from the non-permitted category.

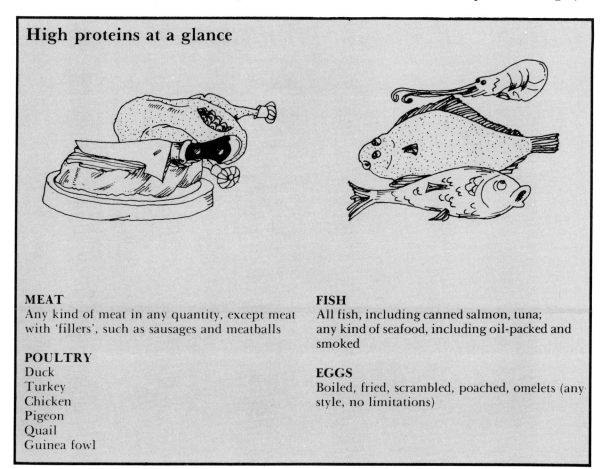

High proteins at a glance

MEAT
Any kind of meat in any quantity, except meat with 'fillers', such as sausages and meatballs

POULTRY
Duck
Turkey
Chicken
Pigeon
Quail
Guinea fowl

FISH
All fish, including canned salmon, tuna;
any kind of seafood, including oil-packed and smoked

EGGS
Boiled, fried, scrambled, poached, omelets (any style, no limitations)

Permitted foods

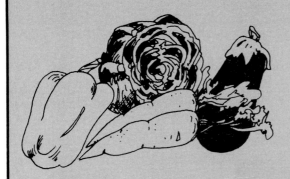

VEGETABLES
Asparagus
Aubergines
Avocados
Bamboo shoots
Beans (French and runner)
Bean sprouts
Broccoli
Brussels sprouts
Cabbage
Cauliflower
Celery
Chicory
Chinese cabbage
Chives
Courgettes
Cucumber
Endive
Fennel
Kale
Kohlrabi
Lettuce
Marrow
Mushrooms
Onions
Parsley
Peppers
Radishes
Spinach
Tomatoes
Turnip
Watercress

GARNISHES FOR SALADS
Anchovies
Chopped fried bacon
French dressing
Grated cheese
Chopped, hard-boiled eggs
Chopped mushrooms (cooked or raw)
Olives (green or black)
Pickles (sour or dill)
Sour cream

FATS
(Fats have no carbohydrates.)
Butter
Margarine
Oil
Lard
Mayonnaise (sugar-free)

CHEESE
125 g (4 oz) a day of any hard, aged cheese

CREAM
(Cream has less carbohydrate than milk. Use it instead of milk.)
20 ml (4 teaspoons) a day of double cream

DESSERTS
Jellies, non-sugar
Sorbets, non-sugar

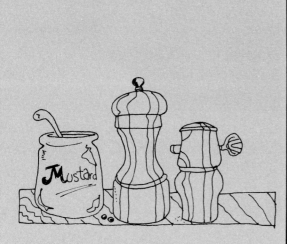

CONDIMENTS
Salt
Pepper
Mustard
Horseradish
Vinegar
Vanilla
Artificial sweeteners
Powdered spices, containing no sugar

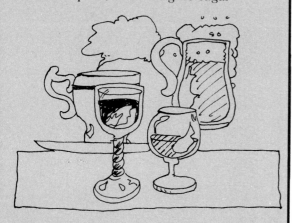

DRINKS
Water
Mineral water
Sugar-free diet soda
Beef or chicken broth
Bouillon
Coffee
Tea

Not permitted
Alcohol
Baked beans
Bananas
Beans (except French and runner)
Biscuits
Bread
Cake
Cashew nuts
Cereal
Cheese spread
Chewing gum
Chocolate
Cornflour
Dates
Figs
Fishcakes
Flour
Fruit, dried
Honey
Ice-cream
Jam
Meatballs
Milk
Pancakes
Pasta
Pastry
Peas
Pickles, sweet
Potatoes
Potatoes, sweet
Relish, sweet
Rice
Sausages
Sugar
Sweets
Syrup
Yogurt, sweetened

Sample Menus

Breakfast This consists mainly of egg dishes, fried, boiled, scrambled or poached, but canned, cooked or fresh fish can be added for variety. The main problem is to find an effective substitute for bread. All crispbreads contain some carbohydrate and 'diet' rolls are a poor substitute. It is important to eat a good breakfast to 'boost' the protein fires to burn off the fat. A high protein bread recipe has been invented as a bread substitute that contains virtually no carbohydrate. It can be rather tricky to make, but it is an effective alternative for those who feel they cannot survive a day without bread.

High Protein Bread

12 SLICES   total weight—10.5 g
           weight per slice—0 9 g

2 eggs at room temperature, separated
¼ teaspoon cream of tartar
2 tablespoons cottage cheese
2 tablespoons soya powder

Preheat the oven to 170°C (325°F), gas mark 3. Set aside a small loaf tin, 15 x 8.5 x 5 cm (6 x 3½ x 2 in).

Beat the egg yolks with a fork. Set aside.

Beat the egg whites with the cream of tartar, using a wire whisk or hand electric beater, so they are very evenly beaten. Beat steadily until the whites are stiff. Fold in the cottage cheese and the egg yolks.

Sift the soya powder gradually and evenly over the egg mixture. Lightly fold it in.

Spoon the mixture into the loaf tin and bake for 30 minutes. Reduce the oven temperature to 150°C (300°F), gas mark 2 and bake for a further 30 minutes, or until the loaf is firm to the touch.

Turn the loaf out on to a wire rack to cool completely. When cold slice into 12 slices.

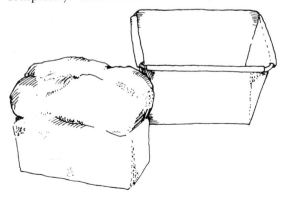

Lunches and snack meals

Start each meal with clear soup, or beef or yeast extract.

MONDAY

Cold meats, or leftover roast meat, served with mixed salad (lettuce, endive, cucumber, tomato) and sugar-free dressings.

TUESDAY

Curried Eggs
SERVES 2

3 eggs, hard-boiled and shelled
1 tablespoon salad cream or mayonnaise
1 tablespoon curry powder
salt and pepper

Cut the eggs in half lengthwise and scoop out the yolk. Reserve the white 'shells'.

Mash the yolks with the salad cream or mayonnaise, the curry powder and salt and pepper to taste.

Transfer the mixture to the scooped out whites. Serve with lettuce and tomato.

WEDNESDAY

Spinach and Cheese Omelets
SERVES 2

1 tablespoon vegetable oil
1 garlic clove, peeled and finely chopped
450 g (1 lb) spinach, washed and chopped
4 eggs, lightly beaten
1 tablespoon water
salt and pepper
1 tablespoon butter
4 tablespoons grated cheese

Heat the vegetable oil in a medium-sized frying-pan. Fry the garlic for 2-3 minutes, or until it is brown. Add the chopped spinach and cook in the oil for a minute.

Meanwhile, beat the eggs and water together with salt and pepper to taste. Melt half the butter in an omelet pan. Add half the eggs, stir and cook for 2-3 minutes or until the omelet is ready.

Add half the spinach and garlic mixture. Sprinkle over half the cheese and fold the omelet over. Cook the second omelet in the same way.

THURSDAY

Scrambled Eggs with Ham
SERVES 2

4 eggs, lightly beaten
salt and pepper
1 tablespoon butter
4 slices cooked ham
150 ml (¼ pint) cream

Preheat the oven to 180°C (350°F), gas mark 4.

Beat the eggs with salt and pepper to taste. Melt the butter in a small saucepan. Add the eggs and cook, stirring constantly, for 3-5 minutes, or until just set. Divide the scrambled eggs equally between the ham slices and roll up.

Arrange the ham rolls in an ovenproof baking dish and pour over the cream.

Bake for 10-15 minutes, or until the cream is bubbling.

Serve with raw vegetables tossed in a French dressing.

FRIDAY

Grilled fish
Any fresh or tinned fish cooked to a traditional recipe and served with zero carbohydrate vegetables.

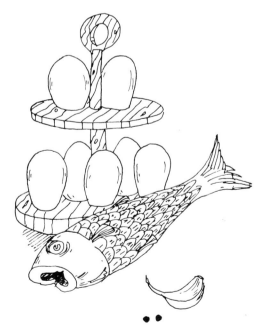

SATURDAY

Caesar Salad
SERVES 2

1 garlic clove, halved
1 lettuce, washed, shaken dry and shredded
4 tablespoons olive oil
2 tablespoons white wine vinegar
1 teaspoon French mustard
salt and pepper
4 slices bacon, rinds removed, grilled
  until crisp and crumbled
1 onion, peeled and chopped
2 tablespoons grated cheese
1 tablespoon chopped, fresh parsley or chives
2 eggs, hard-boiled, shelled and sliced

Rub the inside of a medium-sized bowl with the cut sides of the garlic. Put the lettuce in the bowl and set aside.

Beat together the oil, vinegar, mustard and salt and pepper to taste. Pour over the lettuce and toss to coat thoroughly. Transfer to plates and top with the bacon, onion, cheese and chopped parsley or chives. Decorate with the egg slices.

SUNDAY

Vegetable Delight
SERVES 2

450 g (1 lb) fresh vegetables from zero
  carbohydrate list
1 teaspoon salt
125 g (4 oz) mushrooms, sliced
2 eggs, hard-boiled, shelled and sliced
4 tablespoons grated cheese

Half-fill a large saucepan of water and bring to the boil. Chop the vegetables and add to the water. Stir in the salt. Cook, stirring constantly, for 1 minute.

Strain the vegetables and transfer to a heat-proof serving dish.

Preheat the grill to high. Add the mushrooms to the dish and garnish with the eggs. Sprinkle over the grated cheese.

Grill for 5-8 minutes, or until brown. Serve immediately.

Main Meals

Start with hors d'oeuvres, soups or anti-pasta, using zero carbohydrate foods.

MONDAY

Barbecue-style Chicken
SERVES 2

2 tablespoons water
1 tablespoon Worcestershire sauce
1 tablespoon chilli sauce
1 tablespoon mushroom ketchup
pinch of dry mustard
1 garlic clove, crushed
1 teaspoon horseradish sauce
2 chicken quarters
1 tablespoon butter

Thoroughly combine the water, Worcestershire sauce, chilli sauce, mushroom ketchup, mustard, garlic and horseradish sauce in a large shallow dish. Add the chicken pieces and set aside, turning occasionally, for 10 hours, or overnight, to marinate.

Put the chicken and marinade in a large saucepan and bring to the boil. Cover and simmer for 15 minutes, or until tender.

Melt the butter in a large frying-pan. Add the chicken quarters and fry for 5-7 minutes, or until lightly browned and cooked through.

Serve immediately with hot vegetables from the zero carbohydrate list.

TUESDAY

Pot Roast
Traditionally cooked pot roast served with zero carbohydrate vegetables.

WEDNESDAY

Veal Piccata
SERVES 2

4 slices bacon, rinds removed and chopped
4 tablespoons grated Parmesan cheese
2 eggs, lightly beaten
350 g (12 oz) sliced frying veal
2 tablespoons vegetable oil
2 teaspoons finely grated lemon rind
4 slices lemon

Preheat the oven to 170°C (325°F), gas mark 3.

Fry the bacon for 5 minutes, or until it is cooked. Drain on kitchen paper towels.

Mix together the bacon and Parmesan cheese on a shallow plate. Put the beaten eggs on a separate, shallow plate. Dip the slices of veal into the beaten egg and then into the bacon and cheese mixture to coat them thoroughly.

Heat the oil in a large frying-pan and fry the veal for 5-6 minutes on each side, or until it is evenly browned.

Transfer the veal to a shallow, ovenproof dish and sprinkle over the lemon rind. Arrange the lemon slices on top.

Cover with foil and bake for 30-35 minutes, or until the veal is tender.

Serve with salad or cooked, low carbohydrate vegetables.

THURSDAY

Steak
A medium-sized steak cooked in any way and served with salad.

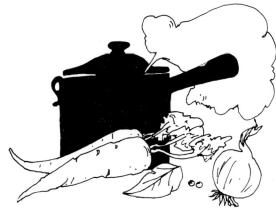

FRIDAY

Trout with Prawns or Shrimps
SERVES 2

2 tablespoons butter
2 tablespoons finely chopped, fresh parsley
2 trout, cleaned
125 g (4 oz) shelled prawns or shrimps
juice of 1 lemon

Preheat the grill to medium.

Mash together the butter and parsley. Spread the parsley butter over the fish.

Grill, turning occasionally, for 12-15 minutes, or until the flesh flakes easily.

Sprinkle the prawns or shrimps and the lemon juice over the trout. Grill for a further 2 minutes, adding extra butter, if necessary.

Serve with lightly-cooked cauliflower and spring beans.

SATURDAY

Roast Lamb or Pork Chops with Chinese-style Vegetables
SERVES 2

2 pork chops or
4 small lamb chops
2 tablespoons vegetable oil
½ small cabbage, finely chopped
4 leeks, finely chopped
1 tablespoon water

Preheat the oven to 180°C (350°F), gas mark 4.

Brush the chops with half the oil and arrange in a roasting tin.

Roast the chops, turning and basting them occasionally, for 30 minutes, or until they are cooked through and tender. Keep them warm.

Heat the remaining oil in a large saucepan. Add the cabbage and leeks. Cook, stirring and tossing constantly, for 1 minute.

Remove the pan from the heat and add the water. Cover and cook for 3 minutes.

Serve immediately with the chops.

SUNDAY

Roast Chicken
Serve with low carbohydrate vegetables, traditionally cooked.

Desserts

Desserts are difficult areas with high protein dieting. Sugar-free jellies are available, but most fruits contain forbidden carbohydrates. Gelatine can be made into desserts flavoured with sugar-free cordials. Cream is allowed.

High protein desserts rely heavily on egg dishes, savouries and sugar-free sorbets. Here is a collection of high protein desserts for high days and holidays. They can be stored in the refrigerator for subsequent use.

Chocolate Mousse
SERVES 8

1 tablespoon cocoa powder
575 ml (1 pint) double cream
15g (½ oz) gelatine
1 tablespoon water
4 teaspoons artificial sweetener
1 teaspoon vanilla essence
25 g (1 oz) chopped walnuts
2 egg whites

Beat together the cocoa and half the cream until the cocoa has dissolved. Set aside.

Half-fill a small saucepan with water and bring to the boil.

Sprinkle the gelatine over the 1 tablespoon of water in a small, heatproof bowl and set aside for 5 minutes to soften.

Set the bowl over the pan of boiling water and cook, stirring constantly, for 3-5 minutes, or until the gelatine has dissolved.

Remove the bowl from the heat and set aside to cool.

Beat the remaining cream with 2 teaspoons sweetener and the vanilla essence until the cream forms soft peaks. Fold in the walnuts. Set aside.

Beat together the egg whites and remaining sweetener until they form stiff peaks.

Fold the cocoa mixture into the cream mixture. Then fold the cocoa and cream mixture into the egg whites. Add more sweetener, if necessary.

Spoon the mixture into a serving dish and chill for 4 hours before serving.

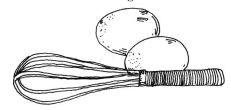

Cheesecake

SERVES 12

225 ml (8 fl oz) double cream
225 g (8 oz) cream cheese, beaten
40 g (1½ oz) gelatine
50 ml (2 fl oz) water
2 eggs, separated
3 tablespoons vanilla essence
juice and grated rind of ¼ lemon
artificial sweetener to taste
pinch of ground cinnamon

Combine 50 ml (2 fl oz) of the cream and the cream cheese in a medium-sized saucepan. Cook gently, stirring constantly, for 5 minutes, or until the cheese has melted. Set aside.

Half-fill a small saucepan with water and bring to the boil.

Sprinkle the gelatine over the water in a small, heatproof bowl and set aside for 5 minutes to soften.

Set the bowl over the pan of boiling water and cook, stirring constantly, for 3-5 minutes, or until the gelatine has dissolved.

Beat the gelatine into the cheese mixture and set aside to cool to room temperature.

Stir the egg yolks, vanilla essence, lemon juice and rind and 4 teaspoons of sweetener into the cheese mixture and set aside.

Beat the remaining cream with a little sweetener until it forms soft peaks. Set aside.

Beat the egg whites until they form stiff peaks. Fold the egg whites into the cream.

Fold the egg and cream mixture into the cheese mixture.

Spoon the mixture into a loose-bottomed cake tin. Sprinkle over the cinnamon. Chill for 2 hours, or until the cake is set.

Vanilla Ice-Cream

SERVES 7

25 g (1 oz) gelatine
275 ml (½ pint) plus 2 tablespoons water
575 ml (1 pint) double cream
artificial sweetener to taste
small pinch of salt
1 tablespoon vanilla essence

Set the thermostat of the refrigerator to its lowest setting.

Half-fill a small saucepan with water and bring to the boil.

Sprinkle the gelatine over 2 tablespoons of water in a small, heatproof bowl and set aside for 5 minutes to soften.

Set the bowl over the pan of boiling water and cook, stirring constantly, for 3-5 minutes, or until the gelatine has dissolved.

Remove the bowl from the heat and set aside to cool.

Pour 275 ml (½ pint) cream and 150 ml (¼ pint) water into a small saucepan. Bring to just below boiling point.

Remove the pan from the heat and stir in the gelatine mixture, sweetener to taste and the salt. Set aside to cool to room temperature.

Stir in the remaining cream, the remaining water and the vanilla essence.

Pour into a freezer tray, cover and freeze for 1 hour.

Turn the mixture into a bowl and beat for 5 minutes, or until smooth.

Return to the freezer tray, cover and freeze until solid.

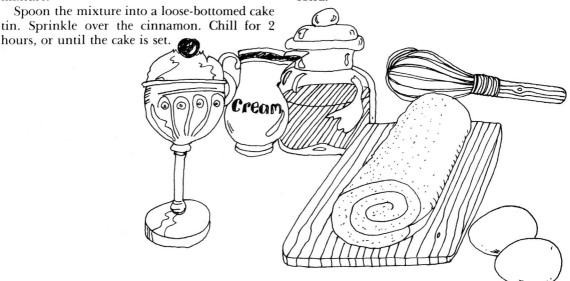

Coffee and Walnut Roll

SERVES 10

8 eggs, separated
pinch of cream of tartar
3 tablespoons instant coffee powder
4 teaspoons vanilla essence
artificial sweetener to taste
25 g (1 oz) chopped walnuts
450 ml (16 fl oz) double cream

Preheat the oven to 190°C (375°F), gas mark 5. Line a swiss roll tin with greaseproof paper and set aside.

Beat the egg whites and cream of tartar together until they form stiff peaks. Set aside.

Stir together the coffee powder and half the vanilla essence until the coffee has dissolved.

Lightly beat the egg yolks. Beat in the coffee and vanilla mixture, sweetener to taste and the walnuts.

Fold the egg yolk mixture into the egg whites.

Spoon the mixture into the prepared tin and spread it evenly with a palette knife.

Bake for 12-15 minutes, or until the top is golden brown.

Meanwhile, cut out a sheet of greaseproof paper slightly larger than the cake tin. Spread it out on a cloth.

Turn the cake out on to the paper and carefully roll it up with the paper wrapped inside it. Hold in position for 2-3 minutes and transfer to a wire rack to cool completely.

Beat the cream with the remaining vanilla extract and sweetener to taste until it forms soft peaks.

Carefully unroll the cake. Spread the cream over it and re-roll, removing the greaseproof paper.

Drinks

Both milk and alcohol are forbidden, except for white wine very occasionally. The body will use alcohol as fuel in preference to protein. Therefore, drinking alcohol lowers protein's specific dynamic action and tends to paralyze slimming.

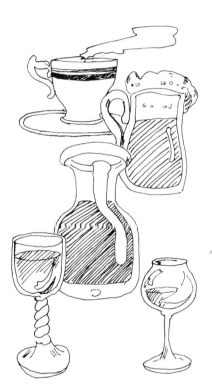

CHAPTER VII

Slim with a friend

Slimming groups follow behavioural techniques to teach their members to eat less. This method has proved both successful and popular. Slimmers may either form their own groups or join one of the existing organizations.

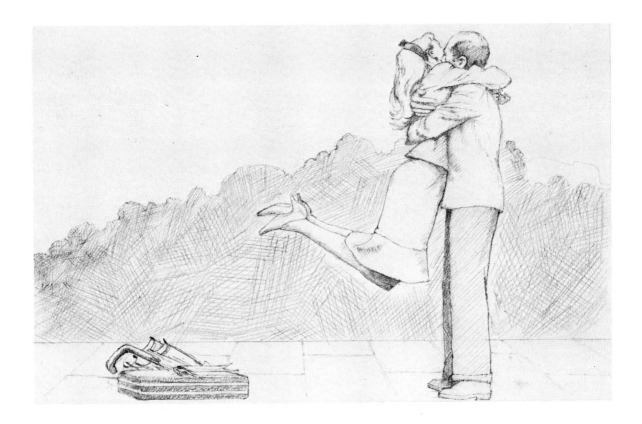

One important part of slimming involves techniques which are called *behavioural*. In a nutshell, these techniques work around the principle of learning to eat less—and feeling good about it. In the history of slimming, behavioural techniques are fairly new—only about 10 years old, in fact. Yet within this period, learned journals have published over 30 reports on how behaviour modification can be effective in slimming and weight-loss.

The technique is partly common sense, relying on the nutritional methods already described in previous chapters. However, special factors are grafted on, such as stimulus control. This is the concept of a special place for eating where *all* food, including snacks, must be consumed.

Slimming groups

Joining a slimming group is an essential part of the behavioural technique. Several slimmers,

who may or may not already be friends, form a slimming group. The leader of the group is very important, although exactly who he or she is can vary from group to group. The leader may be a doctor or nutritionist, but special qualifications are not necessary. Any sensible person with a commitment to helping others lose weight can, with practice, be a group leader. Trials have shown that professional expertise in the group leaders makes little difference, as long as they are sensitive and sensible people, who care about others and who can get into contact with the clients' feelings and fears.

Potential leaders must realize they have a difficult job, perhaps one of the most difficult jobs ever—the changing of lifetime habits. They must also understand that frustration on the part of leader and slimmer is part of the game, which will be a slow, repetitive and drawn-out affair. The leader's power and prestige with the group depends wholly on practical assistance, such as seeking out the frustrations of slimming, when weights 'stick' for instance, and analyzing the cause for the impasse. Leaders who have won their own battle against overweight gain by 'knowing most of the answers'. A good leader can spot the poorly motivated slimmer and either invite her to leave the group or advise her how to make use of a problem to obtain better control of overeating. For example, when someone fears a session of overeating, at Christmas for instance, the impasse can be met by advising alternative activities, such as outings and visits to the theatre. These effectively 'soak up' Christmas fare money, while giving a sense of indulgence at the same time. Leaders must realize that their prime function is to help solve eating problems, not to play psychologist or psychiatrist.

Payment seems to be a motivating factor in the majority of behaviouristic treatments. It seals a contract and must be made in advance. Some groups charge a returnable homework fee as well. This extra sum is given back to the subscriber when all homework tasks are completed. The actual details of the group's finances, the payment of the leader and so on are variable and unimportant to the method of slimming.

Weight Watchers, a prominent, largely behaviouristic, international group, requires a registration fee and a weekly meeting fee, which covers all attendances in that week. It also operates a lifetime membership which, after 'qualification', is free. Many hospitals and health authorities run prepayment behaviouristic schemes, the fees for which vary.

What goes on?

Slimming meetings vary to some extent from group to group, but the following is a typical example and shows you what to expect.

After paying her fee the new slimmer makes a personal commitment to change her weight, with the expectation of hard work. Those who do not make this commitment with enthusiasm usually eliminate themselves from the subsequent programme quite quickly, despite the loss of their pre-paid fees.

During the group discussions, people are not encouraged to analyze the reasons for failure or for not carrying out instructions. This is because discussion of one person's failure tends to reinforce failure in others. Monopolizing or disruptive slimmers are discouraged from dominating the discussion in the group, but they can

air their views privately to the leader afterwards, should they so wish.

Early in group meetings, slimmers are asked to answer a questionnaire and a food diary is also provided.

The first meeting

At the first group meeting, the leader stresses that the organization is not a psychotherapeutic exercise and there will be no sharing of weight or personal information, no humiliations, no testimonials, no praises or admonishments. It is merely a method devoted to learning new eating behaviour and thus losing weight.

Eating questionnaire

Groups may design their own questionnaires, but they should include the following topics: vital identifying information, weight history, brief medical history including drugs taken, and marital history. Weight history questions could be based on these points.

1 Height
2 Present weight
3 Weight pattern (at, say, five-year intervals)
4 Best healthy weight
5 Desired weight-loss
6 Why weight-loss is desired
7 Effect of being overweight on lifestyle and personality
8 Effect of being overweight on others (spouse, children, friends)
9 Past attempts to lose weight (why, when, method, success, failure)
10 Mood changes experienced when losing weight
11 Family weight and medical history (parents, spouse, children)
12 Alcohol consumption per week
13 Amount of exercise taken per day

The diet

Interestingly, no ideal diet is specially recommended or, indeed, necessary and this is stressed by the group leader. Results will be quicker if a slimming diet is accepted, but no mandatory diet is laid down. Some people find this so worrying that some slimming groups give a simple standby system. Weight Watchers base their principles on either the 'free' diet described in Chapter VIII or on the following pattern.

Men and women

BREAKFAST

Fruit, 1 serving:

125 g (4 oz) grapefruit, orange, tangerine, apple puree, blackberries, loganberries, pineapple
or
225 ml (8 fl oz) tomato, vegetable juice *or* 225 g (8 oz) cranberries, strawberries, melon chunks, grapes, cooked rhubarb
or
one of the following: 2 apricots, ½ banana, 10 cherries, ½ grapefruit, 1 orange, 1 peach, 2 plums, 4 prunes, 1 tangerine

Choice of:
1 egg (maximum 4 per week)
or 70 g (2½ oz) soft cheese (maximum 125 g (4 oz) per week)
or 25 g (1 oz) semi-soft *or* hard cheese
or 25 g (1 oz) cereal with ½ milk serving* (maximum 3 servings per week)
or 50 g (2 oz) cooked fish
or 25 g (1 oz) cooked poultry *or* meat (maximum 2-3 servings per day)

Bread, 1 serving **
Beverage, if desired

Women

LUNCH

Choice of:
75-125 g (3-4 oz) cooked poultry, meat *or* fish (visible fat removed)
or 2 eggs
or 150 g (5 oz) soft cheese
or 50 g (2 oz) semi-soft *or* hard cheese
or 175 g (6 oz) cooked pulses (peas, beans, lentils, etc)

125 g (4 oz) green vegetables
Bread, 1 serving **
Beverage, if desired

DINNER

Choice of:
125-175 g (4-6 oz) cooked poultry, meat *or* fish (visible fat removed)
or 225 g (8 oz) cooked pulses (peas, beans, lentils, etc)

125 g (4 oz) green vegetables
Bread, 1 serving ** *if not eaten at lunch-time*
Beverage, if desired

DAILY ALLOWANCE

*Milk: 1 serving=175 ml (6 fl oz) *or* 110 ml (4 fl oz) plain yogurt.
Fats: 1 serving=1 tablespoon margarine, butter, vegetable oil *or* 1 teaspoon mayonnaise.
Fruit: 3 servings per day.
Vegetables: 1 serving=125 g (4 oz).
**Bread: 1 serving=25 g (1 oz) wholemeal bread. If bread is omitted, then 125 g (4 oz) pasta *or* 75 g (3 oz) potato *or* 125 g (4 oz) rice may be substituted.
Beverage: Lemon tea or black coffee.

Men

LUNCH

Choice of:
75-125 g (3-4 oz) cooked poultry, meat *or* fish (visible fat removed)
or 2 eggs
or 150 g (5 oz) soft cheese
or 50 g (2 oz) semi-soft *or* hard cheese
or 175 g (6 oz) cooked pulses (peas, beans, lentils, etc)

125 g (4 oz) green vegetables
Bread, 2 servings **
Beverage, if desired

DINNER

Choice of:
175-225 g (6-8 oz) cooked poultry, meat *or* fish (visible fat removed)
or 350 g (12 oz) cooked pulses (peas, beans, lentils, etc)

125 g (4 oz) green vegetables
Bread, 1 serving **
Beverage, if desired

DAILY ALLOWANCE

*Milk: 1 serving=175 ml (6 fl oz); 2 servings at any time.
Fats: 1 serving=1 tablespoon margarine, butter, vegetable oil *or* 1 teaspoon mayonnaise; 3 servings at mealtimes.
Fruit: 3-5 servings per day.
Vegetables: 1 serving = 125 g (4 oz).
**Bread: 1 serving=25 g (1 oz) wholemeal bread. If bread is omitted, then 125 g (4 oz) pasta *or* 75 g (3 oz) potato *or* 125 g (4 oz) rice may be substituted.
Beverage: Lemon tea or black coffee.

A week of slimming meals

The diet is worked out mainly for women. Asterisks indicate portion variations for men following the diet, and additional foods are given to meet the dietary requirements of men and teenagers.

	MONDAY	TUESDAY	WEDNESDAY	
BREAKFAST	Melon, 1 serving Scrambled egg, 1 Bread, 1 serving Margarine or butter, 1 serving **Teenagers** Add: Milk, 1 serving	Grapefruit juice, 1 serving 25 g (1 oz) hard cheese Enriched white bread, 1 serving Milk, ½ serving	Fruit, 1 serving 25 g (1 oz) cereal Milk, ½ serving **Men and teenagers** Add: Bread, 1 serving	
LUNCH	75-125 g (3-4 oz) fish 125 g (4 oz) peas Lettuce Mayonnaise, 1 serving Fruit, 1 serving **Men and teenagers** Add: Bread, 2 servings	Mushroom omelet (2 eggs) Tossed salad Vegetable oil, 2 servings Bread, 1 serving Fruit, 1 serving Milk, 1 serving **Men and teenagers** Add: Bread, 1 serving	75-125 g (3-4 oz) tuna fish Mayonnaise, 2 servings Celery Asparagus spears, 1 serving Bread, 1 serving Milk, 1 serving Beverage **Men and teenagers** Add: Bread, 1 serving	
SNACK	Milk, 1 serving	Artificially sweetened carbonated beverage	Orange, 1 serving **Teenagers** Add: Milk, 1 serving	
DINNER	125-175 g (4-6 oz) roast turkey* Broccoli, 1 serving Creamed corn, ½ cup Salad Vegetable oil, 1 serving Plain yogurt, 1 serving Fruit, 1 serving *Men 175-225 g (6-8 oz) roast turkey	125-175 g (4-6 oz) baked fish* Cauliflower, 1 serving Heart of lettuce Mayonnaise, 1 serving Fruit, 1 serving Beverage **Men and teenagers** Add: Bread, 1 serving *Men 175-225 g (6-8 oz) baked fish	125-175 g (4-6 oz) hamburger* Carrots, 1 serving Lettuce and tomato salad Vegetable oil, 1 serving Bread, 1 serving Milk, ½ serving Beverage *Men 175-225 g (6-8 oz) hamburger	
SNACK	Tomato juice **Men and teenagers** Add (if desired): Fruit, 1-2 servings **Teenagers** Add (if desired): Milk, 1 serving	Milk, ½ serving **Men and teenagers** Add (if desired): Fruit, 1-2 servings **Teenagers** Add (if desired): Milk, 1 serving	Diet soda **Men and teenagers** Add (if desired): Fruit, 1-2 servings **Teenagers** Add (if desired): Milk, 1 serving	

THURSDAY	FRIDAY	SATURDAY	SUNDAY
75 g (3 oz) cottage cheese Bread, 1 serving Margarine or butter, 1 serving **Teenagers** Add: Milk, 1 serving	Orange juice, 1 serving 25 g (1 oz) cereal Milk, ½ serving Beverage **Men and teenagers** Add: Bread, 1 serving	Tomato juice Poached egg, 1 Bread, 1 serving Margarine or butter, 1 serving Milk, ½ serving	Strawberries, 1 serving 25 g (1 oz) semi-soft cheese Bread, 1 serving Margarine or butter, 1 serving Milk, ½ serving

75 g (3 oz) salami
Mixed green salad
Mayonnaise, 1 serving
Pickle
Bread, 1 serving
Milk, 1 serving
 	
Men and teenagers
Add: Bread, 1 serving
	Grilled cheese sandwich
	  25 g (1 oz) hard cheese,
	  bread, 1 serving
	Pickle
	Shredded cabbage, 1 serving
	Mayonnaise, 1 serving
	
	Men and teenagers
	Add: Bread, 1 serving
	
	Teenagers
	Add: Milk, 1 serving
		75-125 g (3-4 oz) sardines
		Carrots, 1 serving
		Cucumber salad
		Fruit, 1 serving
		Beverage
		
		Men and teenagers
		Add: Bread, 2 servings
		
		Teenagers
		Add: Milk, 1 serving
			75-125 g (3-4 oz) chicken
			125 g (4 oz) beetroot
			Green pepper rings
			Tomato wedges
			Mayonnaise, 1 serving
			Fruit, 1 serving
			Beverage
			
			Men and teenagers
			Add: Bread, 2 servings
			
			Teenagers
			Add: milk, 1 serving

Skimmed milk, 1 serving	Fruit, 1 serving Plain yogurt, 1 serving	Milk, 1 serving	Mixed vegetable juice, 1 serving
125-175 g (4-6 oz) liver* 125 g (4 oz) onions Courgettes, 1 serving Butter, 1 serving Fruit, 1 serving **Men and teenagers** Add: Bread, 1 serving ***Men** 175-225 g (6-8 oz) liver	125-175 g (4-6 oz) roast veal* 75 g (3 oz) baked potato Margarine or butter, 2 servings 125 g (4 oz) Brussels sprouts Fruit, 1 serving Beverage ***Men** 175-225 g (6-8 oz) roast veal	125-175 g (4-6 oz) baked pork chop* Spinach, 1 serving Green salad Mayonnaise, 2 servings Milk, ½ serving Fruit, 1 serving Beverage ***Men** 175-225 g (6-8 oz) baked pork chop	125-175 g (4-6 oz) grilled fish* ½ cup rice Green beans, 1 serving Margarine or butter, 1 serving Milk, ½ serving Fruit, 1 serving Beverage ***Men** 175-225 g (6-8 oz) grilled fish

Fruit, 1 serving
 	
Men and teenagers
Add (if desired):
  Fruit, 1-2 servings
 	
Teenagers
Add (if desired):
  Milk, 1 serving
	Milk, ½ serving
	
	Men and teenagers
	Add (if desired):
	  Fruit, 1-2 servings
	
	Teenagers
	Add (if desired):
	  Milk, 1 serving
		Fruit, 1 serving
		
		Men and teenagers
		Add (if desired):
		  Fruit, 1-2 servings
		
		Teenagers
		Add (if desired);
		  Milk, 1 serving
			Milk, 1 serving
			
			Men and teenagers
			Add (if desired):
			  Fruit, 1-2 servings
			
			Teenagers
			Add (if desired):
			  Milk, 1 serving

What you get for your money

Groups are variable in size but eight to twelve people is ideal. Groups seem to work best if they are comprised of people with very similar problems. For example, people who are 4.5-6.75 kg (10-15 lb) overweight can form one group, while people who are 6.75-13.5 kg (15-30 lb) overweight can form another. It is best to hold meetings around a large table in a comfortable, warm room. Name tags help members to get to know one another. A few basic items of equipment are necessary for some assignments. Group members must have access to good scales. Cheap, bathroom scales are inaccurate and widely variable. If these are all that is available, place them on a hard, uncarpetted surface and mark stand-over footprints clearly on the standing area to give a semblance of correct weight. However, in the 'clinic' proper scales must be available.

A reasonable fee must compensate the group leader for his or her time, and yet be low enough to allow the group to recruit new members. Reasonable course fees range from about £10 to £20 with a similar or smaller returnable 'homework' fee. New members must not be recruited in the middle of the course.

Keeping records

The leader should keep master records, including weekly weighings. These are confidential and are not disclosed to other group members. The weight record is used merely as a tool to measure how eating behaviour is changing. The leader should emphasize the following facts.

1 **Everybody loses and gains weight at his or her own individual rate.**
2 **If daily home weighing is desired, it must always be done at the same time each day, after going to the toilet (voiding urine and faeces). The leader should explain pre-menstrual fluid retention to women.**
3 **Group weight-loss is averaged weekly and privately compared with personal weight-loss.**
4 **Groups may unanimously decide to break confidentiality and share weight-loss experiences, but this should not be suggested to the group by the leader.**

The food diary

At the first meeting new members are introduced to the food diary (see page 87). This will give the

leader the necessary insight into each potential slimmer in order to spot unusual eating patterns, addictions to 'problem foods', 'binge eating' and night-time larder raiders. Agreeing to carry out the rather dull and long-term job of food logging is part of the slimmer's commitment. Some groups invite a non-slimming husband or wife to attend with the slimmer, so that the leader may assess the slimmer's intimate social environment and, perhaps, be ready for 'sabotage' which may subsequently arise in the home. At other groups, spouse involvement only occurs at the end of the course.

Typical meetings

A course usually consists of 10 formal, weekly meetings of 1½ to 2 hours each, including the weigh-in and homework assessment. Individual courses may vary a little but the following summary is fairly typical.

Lesson 1 This is introductory, explains about weigh-ins, how a food diary is kept (see page 87), how the group data sheet and homework credits work (see page 88). Homework for the first week is completion of the food diary and eating place record.

Lesson 2 Weighing details are collected to start group weight graphs, followed by a discussion on how to eliminate the 'cue to eat'. Homework involves the food diary and the keeping of an eating place record.

Lesson 3 After the usual preliminaries of the weigh-in and graph analysis, discussion develops around changing the act of eating, changing places at the table, making food less easily visible, removing serving dishes from sight after serving from them and eating more slowly (more chews per mouthful). Homework includes food diary, record of change in act of eating and elimination of visual food cues at home.

Lesson 4 After the usual preliminaries, the 'behaviour chains' concept is discussed in relationship to 'alternative activities'. The concept of behaviour chains involves making a diary of, for example, how an evening is spent. This might include such entries as (i) eating the evening meal, (ii) sitting down in an easy chair, (iii) watching television, (iv) getting bored with television, (v) feeling sleepy, (vi) going into the kitchen to feed the dog and make coffee, (vii) raiding the biscuit box, (viii) feeling bad about the raid, (ix) wanting more biscuits – and so on. The group explores chain-breaking methods. Homework involves the usual tasks plus puzzling out how to unlink behaviour chains and how to substitute links which, for example, eliminate eating snacks.

Lesson 5 After the usual preliminaries and a discussion of the previous lesson, the slimmer is introduced to specific problem solving and invited to 'be his own therapist'. For example, a large breakfast eater is enjoined to introduce a two minute delay into his meal, not to read the newspaper or listen to the radio while eating, to substitute lower calorie foods, to take smaller portions and to eliminate a favourite breakfast food, such as bacon and eggs. A sensible decision that can (mostly) be kept to is encouraged and the food diary evaluates progress. Homework involves adding to problem solving practices and to continue recording.

Lesson 6 After the usual preliminaries, the lesson is devoted to a review of what has been learned so far and problem solving by group discussion. A concept of pre-planning is introduced; plans are made to take advantage of behaviour modifications which have already been learned and specific foods are planned for pre-selected times and places of eating. Strategies are worked out for parties and slimmers are advised to shop after rather than before a meal to avoid impulse buying of tempting 'goodies'.

Lesson 7 The concepts of smaller plates, leaving some food on the plate and dividing the total meal into two and keeping the second helping in the kitchen are introduced. Eliminating food 'invitations' at the table is stressed, i.e. you ask for everything yourself. Minimizing food contact

where possible is introduced, i.e. only have exactly what is to be eaten on the table. Finally, activity monitoring and recording is added to the regime.

Lesson 8 After the preliminaries, the group is involved in ways of increasing habitual activity. The message is 'increase your normal activities by becoming less efficient'. This means taking the longest route to the shops, leaving the car at the farthest position in the car park, using stairs not lifts and so on. Whenever possible, pedometers are used to record the distance walked. Group members are encouraged to explore the possibilities of activity changes on a progressive scale. Homework now includes completion of food diary, behaviour checklists and activity sheets.

Lesson 9 This needs a calorie counter. After homework has been checked and the traditional weigh-in completed, the process of pre-planning is reviewed and reinforced. The idea is to plan what will be eaten at certain future meals in a habitual way, so that routine replaces decision making in the kitchen. Food cue elimination is also reinforced. External cues to eating are

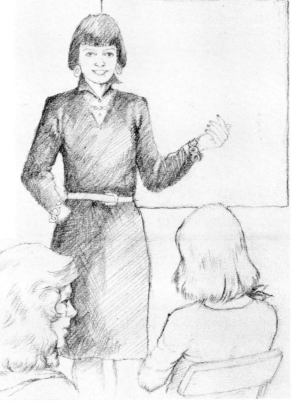

'faded'—the amount left on the plate is increased, no food is offered by others, smaller plates become routine. The whole idea is liberation from childhood eating habits. 'Wasteful' energy spending is further encouraged. Anti-snack tricks are explored—setting a delay before a snack, slow snack eating, limiting snacks to 'eating place' eating, leaving part of snacks uneaten and low calories snacks. Homework now has the extra tasks of finding ways to add 250 'exercise' calories every day for a week and arranging to bring a friend to the group for Lesson 10, in addition to the usual logging of foods, exercise and weight charting.

Lesson 10 This completes the formal course. Cumulative personal and group weight-losses are consolidated, homework is checked and friends are welcomed and told about how the course has worked out. It is stressed that the first nine lessons, although carried out in a group, were, in fact, individual-orientated. Now the social environment is explored. No-one is blamed for the family eating patterns that produce obesity. The only thought is to demonstrate how obesity has occurred. It is stressed that will-power, as such, is not necessary—all that has changed has been behaviour. The basic truth is that *Energy in* (food) always equals *Energy used* (activity) + *Storage* (fat). This can be stated another way:

$$Fat = Food - Activity$$

A short review of the behaviourist principles of weight-loss follows.

1 **Defences against impulse eating.**
2 **How impulses can be 'faded' (delays and time lags).**
3 **Recognition of fattening rationalizations ('someone has to have the biggest portion' and 'if you don't eat well you get ill').**
4 **Capitalization of refusing to eat when not hungry.**
5 **Recognition of bulk fillers.**
6 **Substituting low for high calorie foods, wherever possible.**

The group and the visitors are taken through the course retrospectively, starting with the food diary of Lesson 1 and are reminded that overweight people have learned to become more sensitive to food cues than other people.

After the behavioural basics have been explained to the visitors and revised by the slimmers, the principles of extra calorie-using exercise are explained. An important part of the final get-together is to try to break down stereotyped family interactions that can sabotage the new eating patterns. It is stressed that other people cannot read our minds, so we have to tell them what we want and ask for help and support in changing part of our relationship with them. 'If those around you help you to succeed, then your success is their success' is the message.

The visitors are asked to help with praise, even to experiment themselves with the techniques, to dissociate the idea of affection and sharing from thoughts of food (avoid food gifts), never to offer food at any time and to minimize food topics in conversations. It is also stressed that family entertainment should concentrate on low calorie foods. Snacks should be eaten in private and the whole family join in exercise programmes. The course closes with a pay-back for homework assignments and an invitation to keep in touch for a further five maintenance weeks and to attend the clinic 'free' for five more weeks.

Keeping a food diary

The food diary, introduced in Lesson 1, will be based on the example given opposite. Replies should be simple and consistent.

1 Note the time you started to eat the meal or snack.
2 Note how long you spent eating it.
3 Note whether it was a meal or a snack.
4 Note the type of food and the size of portion. Choose units of measurement that you can use each day, e.g. two potatoes and one slice of meat or 1 tablespoon of potatoes and 25 g (1 oz) of meat. Accuracy is not quite as important as
5 Note how hungry you were before you started to eat.
6 Note your mood immediately before and during eating.
7 Note what else you were doing, e.g. watching television.
8 Note where you had your meal, e.g. kitchen, cafe, in front of the television.
9 Note whether you were eating alone or with others.
10 Note whether you were sitting, standing, walking or lying down.

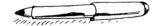

Food diary and eating place record

Name   Day

	Time	Duration	Meal or snack	Food—type and quantity	Degree of hunger	Mood	Other activities	Eating place	Alone or with others	Position
Early morning										
Breakfast										
Morning										
Lunch										
Afternoon										
Dinner										
Evening										
Bedtime										

Homework projects		Checked by	Refund
Lesson 1	Introductory meeting **Homework** Complete food diary		
Lesson 2	How to eliminate the 'cue to eat' **Homework** Complete food diary Complete eating questionnaire		
Lesson 3	How to change eating habits **Homework** Complete food diary Record changes in the act of eating Record elimination of visual food 'cues'		
Lesson 4	Behaviour chains and alternative activities **Homework** Complete food diary Prepare an evening's food and activity diary Suggest chain-breaking methods		
Lesson 5	How to isolate the slimmer's own particular problems **Homework** Complete food diary Suggest ways to solve problems		
Lesson 6	Progress review and pre-planning **Homework** Complete food diary Suggest forward planning strategies Suggest behaviour checklist		
Lesson 7	New strategies to eliminate the 'cue to eat' **Homework** Complete food diary Complete behaviour checklist Monitor and record activity		
Lesson 8	How to increase energy expenditure **Homework** Complete food diary Complete activity sheet Complete behaviour checklist		
Lesson 9	How to establish new routines and change old habits **Homework** Complete food diary Complete activity sheet Complete behaviour checklist Use up an *extra* 250 calories per day in exercise Arrange to bring a friend to next meeting		
Lesson 10	Completion of formal course		

Behaviour checklists

Behaviour checklists should be completed by the slimmer each day. A system of grading the replies is worked out by the group and daily and weekly 'totals' recorded. The slimmer's weight at the end of each week should also be noted. This forms a major part of the behaviour therapy.

Lesson 7

1 Do you avoid eating snacks in the morning?
2 Do you avoid eating snacks in the afternoon?
3 Do you avoid eating snacks in the evening?
4 Do you sometimes change places at the dining table?
5 Do you try to eat your meals in the same room?
6 Do you always put food away in a cupboard?
7 Do you remove serving dishes from the table?
8 Do you eat more slowly?
9 Do you put your knife and fork down between mouthfuls?
10 Do you take more chews per mouthful?
11 Do you make coffee but resist the biscuit?
12 Do you delay before eating a meal?
13 Do you have a meal without listening to the radio?
14 Do you have a meal without reading a newspaper?
15 Do you eat low-calorie foods?
16 Do you take smaller portions?
17 Do you eliminate some favourite fattening foods?
18 Do you plan in advance and prepare a shopping list?
19 Do you shop after a meal?
20 Do you use smaller plates?
21 Do you divide your meal into two halves and keep the second helping in the kitchen?
22 Do you refuse offers of food?
23 Do you eat only what is on the table?

Lesson 9

1 Is contact with food minimized?
2 Is food stored out of sight?
3 Do you eat only what you need?
4 Do you eat more slowly?
5 Do you avoid other activities while eating, such as listening to the radio or reading a book?
6 Do you walk to the shops by a longer route?
7 Do you leave the car further away from your destination?
8 Do you use stairs not lifts?
9 Do you use an extra 250 calories a day in exercise?
10 Do you plan meals in advance?
11 Do you leave food on the plate?
12 Do you always use smaller plates?
13 Do you refuse food offered by others?
14 Do you pause before eating a snack?
15 Do you eat your snack slowly?
16 Do you limit snack eating to the eating place?
17 Do you leave part of your snack uneaten?
18 Do you eat low-calorie snacks?
19 Do you find alternative activities to eating?
20 Do you talk less about food?

Activity sheet – Lesson 9

Fill in the total time spent walking each day and minutes of exercise or *extra* activities. Work out the number of 'exercise' calories spent. The target is 250 *extra* calories per day.

	MONDAY		TUESDAY		WEDNES.		THURS.		FRIDAY		SAT.		SUNDAY	
	Mins	Cals	Mins	Cals	Mins	Cals	Mins	Cals	Mins	Cals	Mins	Cals	Mins	Cals
Walking														

Exercise calorie counter – Lesson 9
(10 minutes continuous activity)

| Weight kg | 57 | 68 | 79 | 91 | 102 | 113 | 125 | 136 |
lb	125	150	175	200	225	250	275	300
Assembly line and light factory work	20	25	30	30	35	40	45	50
Badminton	55	60	65	75	85	95	105	115
Basketball	75	80	85	95	105	115	130	140
Boxing	120	130	150	175	190	215	235	255
Bricklaying	30	35	40	45	50	55	60	65
Carpentry	35	40	45	50	60	65	70	80
Car repair	35	40	50	55	60	70	75	85
Chopping wood	65	75	85	95	100	120	135	155
Cycling (fast)	90	110	125	140	160	180	195	215
Cycling (leisurely)	40	50	60	65	75	85	90	100
Dancing (ballroom)	30	40	50	55	60	70	75	85
Dancing (disco)	60	65	70	75	85	95	105	115
Football	80	90	100	110	125	135	150	165
Gardening (light)	30	35	40	45	50	60	65	75
General housework	35	40	50	55	60	70	75	80
Golf	40	40	45	55	60	70	75	85
Jogging	90	110	125	140	160	180	195	215
Judo	115	130	150	175	190	215	235	255
Karate	115	130	150	175	190	215	235	255
Light office work	25	30	35	40	45	50	55	60
Making beds	35	40	45	50	60	65	75	85
Mowing (manual)	40	45	55	60	65	75	80	85
Mowing (power)	35	40	50	55	60	65	75	80
Riding	55	65	80	90	100	110	125	135
Road repair and heavy work	60	70	80	90	100	110	120	130

| Weight kg | 57 | 68 | 79 | 91 | 102 | 113 | 125 | 136 |
lb	125	150	175	200	225	250	275	300
Running	120	140	165	185	210	230	255	280
Running on the spot	200	240	285	325	365	405	445	490
Sitting (talking)	15	20	20	25	30	30	35	35
Sitting (television or reading)	10	10	15	15	20	20	20	25
Sitting (writing)	15	15	20	25	30	30	35	35
Skiing (alpine)	80	95	115	130	145	160	175	195
Skiing (water)	65	75	90	105	115	130	140	165
Sleeping	10	10	15	15	20	20	20	25
Snow clearing	70	80	90	100	115	130	145	160
Standing still	10	15	15	20	20	25	25	30
Sprinting	165	195	230	260	295	325	360	395
Sweeping leaves	50	60	70	80	90	100	110	120
Swimming	70	90	100	110	120	130	140	150
Table tennis	40	40	45	50	60	65	70	80
Tennis	60	65	80	90	105	115	125	135
Volleyball	60	65	70	75	85	95	105	115
Walking -3 kph (2 mph)	30	35	40	45	55	60	65	70
Walking downstairs	60	65	75	90	100	110	120	135
Walking upstairs	150	175	200	230	260	290	320	350
Washing/dressing	25	30	40	40	45	55	60	65
Washing (floors)	40	45	55	60	70	75	85	90
Washing (windows)	35	40	50	55	60	70	75	85
Weeding	50	60	70	80	90	100	110	120
Wrestling	115	130	150	175	190	215	235	255

The Van Itallie cure

The Van Itallie 'cure' is another example of several behaviourist slimming treatments which involve group discussion and also a knowledge of the calorific values of food. In practice, it is reinforced by exercise regimes. The core of the 'cure' is an eating recording exercise. After each meal, the slimmer completes charts which record the following details.

1 **Duration of eating in minutes (hunger fades with time taken eating).**
2 **Place of eating.**
3 **Physical position (at table, in armchair).**
4 **Company while eating.**
5 **Associated activity (alone, watching television, listening to the radio).**
6 **Mood (neutral, bored, tense, angry, rushed).**
7 **Degree of hunger (none, mild, extreme).**
8 **Type of food eaten (full description of menu).**
9 **Total calorific intake.**
10 **Techniques, if any, embodied into meal to reduce weight.**

The diet works only when the calories expended outstrip the calories taken. Writing down meal profiles (the script) acts as a realistic reinforcement of the personal slimming contract. Looking at the script at regular meetings of the slimming group provides subjects for discussion.

An interesting aspect of this slimming technique is that it arouses a feeling of contempt for the way food dominates the slimmer's lifestyle. Food and its relentless logging take up a disproportionate amount of time and attention. Van Itallie dieters put food in its proper place and stress that the jotting down of every meal to the last calorie is extremely boring. If you have to record each snack in detail, you tend to stop eating them. Simple meals are more easily described than elaborate *haute cuisine*. Total calorie reduction can be sudden (reducing to 1,500 calories a day) to produce rapid weight-loss. Exercise should be gradually increased.

There is really no need to go to a special slimming clinic to exploit this useful 'cure'. A few, interested overweight friends can set up a self-help group themselves.

Does it work?

How far does the extended commitment of the behaviouristic type of dieting pay slimming dividends? Until quite recently, many nutritionists interested in slimming techniques have only paid lip-service to its use. Yet examples of the successful commercial use of behaviouristic principles are not hard to find. Most restaurateurs, particularly those who run 'eat as much as you like', self-service establishments quickly realized the cost-effectiveness of small plates. Even at *haute cuisine* restaurants or at banquets, the smaller the plate, the more easily satisfied is the customer, who refuses proferred vegetable helpings, not because he or she does not want them, but because a heaped plate looks so greedy and inelegant. Such portion control in action on a large scale often adds dramatically to commercial profitability.

News of a more factual and scientific nature slipped into the world's medical literature, almost unnoticed, in late 1980. The British medical journal, *The Lancet*, reported a controlled trial of behaviour therapy, drug therapy and their combination in the treatment of 120 obese women and 10 obese men over a six month period of treatment. Furthermore, and this is very important, their weights one year later were also analyzed in this study. The results of this study inclined many doctors and nutritionists interested in the science of slimming towards behaviour therapy.

Most of the volunteers recruited for the study were middle-aged and over half of the women were housewives. To try to assess the effects of behavioural slimming, the potential slimmers were divided into three treatment groups and two control groups. They were all asked to keep to a 1,000-1,200 calorie diet. One group received straightforward behaviour therapy like that described earlier in this chapter. A second group was treated with the appetite suppressant drug fenfluramine. The third treatment group received both behaviour therapy and appetite suppressant treatment. The first control group was a 'queue' group for inclusion in subsequent behaviour type programmes. The second control group, which was termed the 'doctor's office medication' group, was given average medical advice on obesity. This included fenfluramine, reducing diets, exercise regimes, advice on health and encouragement.

Initially, the group treated with fenfluramine enjoyed a greater weight-loss than the behaviour therapy group. However, at the end of a year, behaviour therapy 'won' outright on permanent weight-loss. Strangely, perhaps, volunteers who received behaviour therapy plus slimming pill therapy did rather poorly in comparison.

CHAPTER VIII

Other popular diets

This chapter examines several diets which have large followings in Europe and the United States and it explains their success. The dietary principles are discussed and the advantages and disadvantages analyzed.

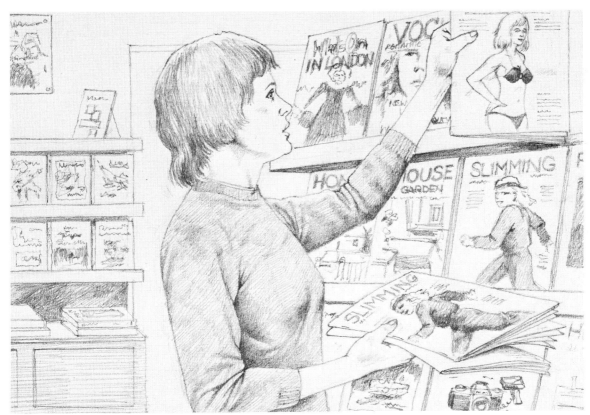

One way to be noticed in the sometimes heady world of dieting and nutrition is to be attacked by the medical establishment. Often, the more vehemently a diet is criticized by the pillars of the establishment, the more the press and the public prick up their ears and open their eyes. 'Is there', they seem to ask, 'something here orthodox doctors don't know or would like to keep quiet?'. In the United States the American Medical Association is the supreme body of the medical establishment. So Dr Robert C. Atkins achieved overnight fame when the AMA made charges against the Atkins' diet on the grounds of 'the possibilities of various results and (ill) effects'. With the organization of an enquiry by the U.S. Senate Select Committee on Nutrition and Human Needs, Dr Atkins' fame was virtually assured and his book, *Dr Atkins' Diet Revolution*, rapidly went through 34 printings.

What is the Atkins' Diet?

Is there very much to be said in support of Dr Atkins' claim that his diet can help the obese to lose weight fairly easily, with a reasonable expectation of success and a high degree of safety?

It would seem, on examination, that there is.

In effect, the Atkins' Diet is a high protein (high fat) diet that involves no calorie counting. Very little carbohydrate is allowed. Dr Atkins points out that no pills are necessary because you are 'never hungry, you eat luxuriously' (if rather expensively) 'and you lose weight and inches rapidly'. What is more, 'no one even knows you're dieting'.

Why is it different?

The Atkins' Diet differs from others in a number of ways, for it is worked out around a system that might be called 'ketosis control'. (Ketosis occurs when there is an acute lack of carbohydrate in the diet. Fat then becomes 'stuck' at an incomplete metabolic stage. See Chapter I for further details.) The presence or absence of ketosis is easily monitored by testing the urine for substances called ketones. This can be done simply by dipping a medicated slip of paper, called a Ketostix, into a fresh specimen of urine. If the test paper goes purple, then ketones are present in the urine in some quantity, indicating the successful 'burning up' of body fat.

Ketostix is easily obtained from chemists and was invented as an aid to diabetic management and diagnosis, as the presence of ketones in the urine of a person on a normal diet is an indication of the disease. Using the Ketostix to monitor fat breakdown in normal, non-diabetic people is the essence of the Atkins' method of dieting.

Getting down to details

You should obtain your doctor's approval before starting the Atkins' Diet. It has five stages.

Stage 1 During this stage, usually five to seven days, you must eat absolutely no carbohydrate. Dr Atkins insists that no slimming pills or diuretics (water pills or injections) are given. He also sensibly advises a daily multivitamin dose for all dieters, supplementary calcium tablets if leg cramps occur, or potassium supplements if undue fatigue is manifested.

All foods eaten during these days must be carefully listed. Permitted foods are all meats, fish, poultry, eggs, cheese, mixed salads and clear soups. Zero calorie drinks, such as sodas, black coffee and lemon tea, are unrestricted. Only carbohydrate-free rolls are allowed and bread and crispbread are banned. Alcohol is also forbidden. Dr Atkins advises a Ketostix test after five days. On this strict regime, the Ketostix turns purple, showing a well marked ketosis quite quickly. If this is not the case, take the salads out of the diet or retest in two days.

Stage 2 During this stage, a little carbohydrate should be added to the diet ('those that you missed most', as Dr Atkins puts it). If the Ketostix still turns purple a few days later, a little more carbohydrate is allowed. In this way you can find what Dr Atkins calls your *critical carbohydrate level*, the point at which the urine test stick no longer turns purple. This is countered by again reducing the carbohydrates until a constant or very nearly constant purple Ketostix is maintained daily.

Dr Atkins stresses that, to begin with, Ketostix testing should be carried out at varying times of day. This is because ketosis increases and decreases with food intake and activity. Once you have established when the deepest purple reaction occurs, continue to test at this time.

Stage 3 Provided ketosis is maintained, more vegetables can be added to the diet and possibly,

even an alcoholic drink. If the Ketostix does not turn purple when the urine is tested, return to the previous stage.

Stage 4 Fruit is added to the diet at this stage and half a slice of bread or toast is allowed. It is essential to maintain at least a lavender coloured tinge to the Ketostix throughout the gradual upstaging of the diet. You must keep a dietary diary all the time, to note and, if necessary, modify carbohydrate intake.

Stage 5 Dr Atkins describes this stage as 'bending the diet without breaking it'. Foods can be added, without Ketostix control, until weight-loss slows to less than 450 g (1 lb) a week. Emphasis is now on maintaining an ideal weight. Dr Atkins stresses that 'the main change that has to be made is in your head'. Many obese people simply cannot eat what others do and stay thin, probably due to an inborn, metabolic defect. Their bodies do not handle food in the same way as that of Mr Constant Weight, so life-long control is necessary. Dr Atkins advises his dieters to set themselves a 2.5 kg (5 lb) ideal weight range and, if necessary, to go back and flip from stage to stage in his diet schedules to keep that way. He advises such people to make a choice of carbohydrates to which they should adhere for the rest of their lives and to eschew sweets and sugars forever. He claims that sweets and starches can be as addictive as drugs or cigarettes and this addiction must be mastered by an accepted denial of such substances.

Is it safe and effective?

The verdict on Dr Atkins' Diet seems to be that, despite the fears of the medical establishment, controlled and monitored ketosis is a safe and effective method of slimming for normal people. It does not, as was initially suggested, make the dieter prone to anorexia (loss of appetite) nor does it affect the kidneys. Dr Atkins claims, with justification, that if a doctor has any doubts as to whether or not a slimmer should use his diet, then he should test for kidney function and blood lipid levels. One matter of anxiety to the AMA was Dr Atkins' claim that his diet was suitable for pregnant women. He stands by his statement that 'there exists not one shred of evidence that this diet causes any maternal of foetal complication'. This claim has not been refuted by the medical profession.

The Scarsdale Medical Diet

About 20 years ago, Dr Herman Tarnower, an American physician, founded a new medical centre devoted to weight control. Widely experienced in general practice and cardiology, he decided, in contrast to some of his competitors, to win over rather than to antagonize his fellow physicians. His best selling book, *The Complete Scarsdale Medical Diet plus Dr Tarnower's Lifetime Keep Slim Program*, was dedicated to 'the American medical profession which has contributed so much help and comfort to all mankind'. Both his overtures and his style have kept medical opinion reasonably favourable, although ketosis, which he calls 'fast fat metabolism', is part and parcel of his diet.

The Scarsdale diet has probably been the most popular 'new' diet of the past ten years. It owes its popularity to its efficiency and its variety. The persuasive powers of its original protagonist have also contributed to its worldwide success.

The Scarsdale diet is a modification of the high protein diets described in Chapter VI. It more than triples the amount of protein taken compared with normal dietary intake (43 per cent protein compared with 10-15 per cent). Fat intake, however, is cut by half (from 40-45 per cent to 22.5 per cent). Carbohydrate intake is also cut by about 50 per cent. These modifications to the diet must be strictly adhered to during the reducing period. This rather punitive regime is alternated every two weeks with more generous eating. Once the slimmer's weight approaches normality, however, he proceeds to a 'Keep Trim' eating style.

The Scarsdale dietary system answers many of the classical questions raised by potential, and perhaps unconvinced, slimmers. For instance, the question 'How can I afford all the chops and steaks on your diet?' brought about the Money Saver modification of the Scarsdale principle. 'What do I do if I want to entertain or eat out?' produced the Gourmet Diet. Overweight travellers, who find the diets boring and too 'American' can enjoy the International Diet well seasoned with Japanese, French, Italian, Greek and Spanish cookery. Eventually, even a Vegetarian Scarsdale Diet was developed.

One of the most attractive features of the Scarsdale plan is that it takes the depression out of dieting. It is also a good diet for the type of person who likes to follow a set of clear instructions. If this description fits you and you are also willing to monitor progress, or lack of it, on charts, the chances are that Dr Tarnower's approach to slimming is right for you.

How it works

The Scarsdale Diet is really two diets in one. The first is the *Scarsdale Medical Diet*, (SMD), during which weight is shed for two weeks. This is followed by the *Keep Trim Programme* for two weeks. Then, if you need to lose more weight, you return to the original SMD regime for a further fortnight.

Weight charting is part of the process and is simplicity itself. Weigh yourself, preferably without clothes, every morning and record the weight on a table (see page 102).

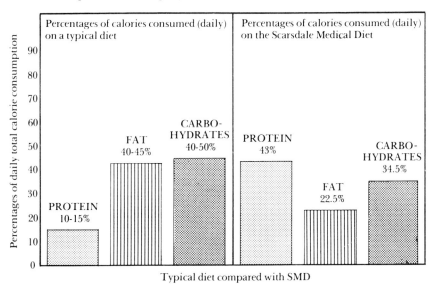

Typical diet compared with SMD

The basic Scarsdale rules

1 Eat exactly what is assigned. Do not substitute.
2 Do not drink any alcoholic drinks.
3 Eat only carrots and celery, if you eat between meals, but you may have as much as you wish.
4 The only beverages allowed are black coffee (ordinary or decaffeinated), tea, soda water (with lemon, if desired) and diet sodas in any flavour. You may drink as often as you wish.
5 Prepare all salads without oil, mayonnaise or other rich dressings. Use only lemon and vinegar.
6 Do not add butter, margarine or other fats to vegetables. You may add lemon juice.
7 All meat should be very lean. Remove all visible fat before eating. Remove skin and fat from chicken and turkey before eating.
8 It is not necessary to eat everything listed, but do not substitute or add.
9 Lunch and dinner interchangeable.
10 A substitute lunch is suggested.
11 Never overload your stomach. Stop eating when you feel full.
12 Do not stay on the Diet for more than fourteen days at a time.

A Scarsdale-type Diet

BREAKFAST (every day)
½ grapefruit or similar quantity of raw fruit without sugar
1 slice of toasted High Protein Bread*
Coffee or tea (no sugar, cream or milk)

	MONDAY	TUESDAY	WEDNESDAY
LUNCH	Assorted lean meats—chicken, turkey, tongue, lean beef Tomatoes Coffee or tea or calorie-free drink	Fruit salad—any combination of fresh fruit Coffee or tea	Tuna fish or salmon salad (oil drained off) with lemon and vinegar dressing Fresh fruit Coffee of tea
DINNER	Fish or shellfish Mixed salad, as many green vegetables as you wish 1 slice of toasted High Protein Bread* Fresh fruit Coffee or tea	Grilled, lean hamburgers Salad made from tomatoes, lettuce, celery, olives or cucumber Coffee or tea	Sliced, roast lamb (all visible fat removed) Salad of lettuce, tomatoes, cucumber, celery Coffee or tea

Substitute Lunch

½ cup low-fat or cottage cheese
1 tablespoon plain yogurt
3 walnuts, shelled and chopped
1 apple or orange, peeled and sliced

Mix together the cheese, cream and chopped nuts. Arrange the fruit slices over the top and serve with tea, coffee (no sugar) or calorie-free soda.

High Protein Bread

1 teaspoon dry yeast
225 ml (8 fl oz) lukewarm water
½ teaspoon salt
1 teaspoon sugar
½ teaspoon cider vinegar
75 g (3 oz) soya flour
25 g (1 oz) gluten flour
150 g (5 oz) wholemeal flour

Sprinkle the yeast over the water and set aside in a warm, draught-free place for 5 minutes.

Stir together the yeast mixture, salt, sugar and vinegar. Sift over the flours and mix together until all the ingredients are thoroughly combined and the dough comes away from the sides of the bowl.

Turn the dough out on to a lightly floured board and knead for 5 minutes, or until it is smooth and elastic.

Shape the dough into a loaf and transfer it to a lightly greased loaf tin. Cover with a damp cloth and set aside in a warm, draught-free place for 2-3 hours, or until the dough has almost doubled in bulk.

Preheat the oven to 170°C (325°F), gas mark 3. Bake the bread for 1 hour, or until well browned and cooked through.

Turn the loaf out on to a wire rack to cool. When cold, the bread may be stored in the refrigerator.

THURSDAY	FRIDAY	SATURDAY	SUNDAY
2 eggs cooked in any style (without using fat) Low-fat cottage cheese Courgettes or green beans or sliced or stewed tomatoes 1 slice of toasted High Protein Bread*	Assorted cheeses Spinach 1 slice of toasted High Protein Bread* Coffee or tea	Fruit salad Coffee or tea	Cold or hot turkey or chicken (skin and visible fat removed) Tomatoes, carrots, cabbage, broccoli or cauliflower Fresh fruit Coffee or tea
Roast, grilled or barbecued chicken (skin and visible fat removed) Spinach, green peppers, green beans Coffee or tea	Fish or shellfish Salad and as many fresh vegetables as desired 1 slice of toasted High Protein Bread* Coffee or tea	Roast turkey or chicken (skin and visible fat removed) Salad of tomatoes and lettuce Fresh fruit Coffee or tea	Grilled steak (all visible fat removed) Salad of lettuce, cucumber, celery, tomatoes Coffee or tea *Recipe for High Protein Bread given above.

97

The Keep Trim Programme

After two weeks on the SMD the next two weeks are spent on the Keep Trim half of the programme, regardless of weight-loss. Again, you should keep a charted day by day record. A new set of rules applies.

Keep trim rules

1 Eat only two slices of **High Protein Bread** a day.
2 No sugar is allowed—sugar substitutes may be used.
3 No potatoes, pasta or similar flour-based foods are permitted.
4 No dairy fats are allowed.
5 Sweets and desserts are forbidden, with the exception of gelatine desserts made without sugar.
6 Up to 43 ml (1½ fl oz) of spirits, OR 128 ml (1½ fl oz) of dry wine, OR 225 ml (8 fl oz) low calorie beer per day is allowed. No ordinary beer or ale is allowed.
7 Carrots and celery may be eaten at any time.

Gourmet recipes

Any recipes from an ordinary cookery book are suitable for the Keep Trim programme, provided those which include frying, cooking in oil or butter, or fat bound sauces are avoided and that the above rules are followed. Dr Tarnower uses psychology to reinforce his message by telling his dieters not to be obsessed with the 'don'ts' of the diet, but rather to use the imagination to explore the 'do's'. Some gourmet recipes follow which are suitable for the Keep Trim programme.

Lunches

American Style Salad
SERVES 1

1 tablespoon gelatine
50 ml (2 fl oz) clear stock
dash chilli sauce
175 g (6 oz) finely chopped vegetables
25 g (1 oz) hard cheese, diced
salt

Sprinkle the gelatine over the stock and cook, stirring constantly, until it has completely dissolved. Stir in the chilli sauce, vegetables, cheese and salt to taste.

Pour the mixture into a mould and set aside to cool to room temperature. Chill in the refrigerator for 1 hour, or until set.

Turn out the mould and serve with lettuce and low calorie dressing.

Spinach Cheese
SERVES 1

1 slice wholemeal bread
150 ml (5 fl oz) water
175 g (6 oz) frozen spinach, thawed
1 egg, lightly beaten
50 g (2 oz) low-fat cheese
1 tablespoon grated Parmesan cheese

Preheat the oven to 190°C (375°F), gas mark 5.

Soak the bread in the water for 10 minutes.

Squeeze the bread gently to remove excess water. Thoroughly mix together the bread and all the remaining ingredients. Pile the mixture into an ovenproof, non-stick dish and bake until lightly browned.

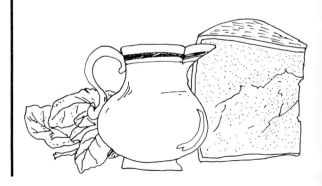

Eggs with Chinese-style Vegetables
SERVES 1

1 teaspoon vegetable oil
1 onion, peeled and chopped
1 garlic clove, crushed
1 tomato, sliced
½ green pepper, seeded and chopped
1 tablespoon clear stock or meat extract
25 g (1 oz) cooked green vegetables, chopped
2 eggs, hard-boiled, shelled and quartered

Heat the oil in a frying-pan. Add the onion, garlic, tomato and pepper and cook, stirring occasionally, for 5-7 minutes, or until the onion is translucent. Stir in the stock or meat extract, the greens and the eggs. Cook, stirring constantly, until the mixture is heated through. Serve immediately.

Marinated Vegetables
SERVES 1

4 small courgettes, sliced and parboiled
50 g (2 oz) cooked green beans
1 green pepper, seeded and chopped
2 cocktail onions
½ lemon, sliced
Marinade:
225 ml (8 fl oz) chicken stock
2 tablespoons dry white wine
2 tablespoons lemon juice
1 garlic clove, crushed
1 tablespoon chopped, fresh parsley
1 teaspoon dried thyme
1 teaspoon Worcestershire sauce
salt

Mix together all the marinade ingredients and simmer for 30 minutes.

Stir in the courgettes, green beans, green pepper, cocktail onions and lemon slices.

Transfer the mixture to a shallow dish, cover with foil and set aside to cool to room temperature. Store in the refrigerator for 2-3 days, or until required.

Stuffed Tomato
SERVES 1

1 large tomato
4 tablespoons cooked rice
40 g (1½ oz) grated cheese
salt and pepper

Preheat the oven to 180°C (350°F), gas mark 4.

Cut a thin slice from the top of the tomato. Scoop out half the tomato pulp and thoroughly mix it with the rice and 25 g (1 oz) of the cheese. Stir in salt and pepper to taste.

Pile the mixture into the tomato shell and sprinkle over the remaining cheese. Place the tomato in an ovenproof dish and bake for 15 minutes.

Prawn or Shrimp Salad
SERVES 1

125 g (4 oz) prawns or shrimps, shelled
1 tablespoon tartar sauce
mixed salad
1 slice High Protein Bread, toasted and cut
   into triangles
1 tablespoon diced melon

Thoroughly mix together the prawns or shrimps and the sauce. Spoon the mixture over the salad and garnish with the toast and melon.

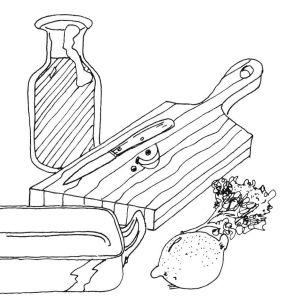

Dinners

Serve the following dishes with low- or zero-carbohydrate vegetables.

Chicken with Tarragon
SERVES 1

1 piece chicken (breast or joint)
110 ml (4 fl oz) chicken stock
2 teaspoons dried tarragon
1 tablespoon dry white wine
1 egg yolk

Put the chicken, half the stock and the tarragon into a medium-sized saucepan. Cover and simmer for 30 minutes.

Remove the chicken from the pan, set aside and keep warm.

Add the remaining stock to the pan and bring to the boil. Remove the pan from the heat and set aside.

Beat together the wine and egg yolk. Pour the mixture into the stock and beat with a wire whisk until the sauce is thick and smooth.

Pour the sauce over the chicken and serve immediately, with braised celery slices.

Veal Escalope
SERVES 1

125 g (4 oz) veal escalope, pounded thin
1 garlic clove, crushed
¼ teaspoon pepper
½ teaspoon salt
1 teaspoon vegetable oil
1 tablespoon chopped lean bacon
50 ml (2 fl oz) tomato juice
1 tablespoon capers
50 ml (2 fl oz) dry white wine

Rub the veal on both sides with the garlic, pepper and salt and set aside.

Heat the oil in a frying-pan. Add the veal and cook for 2 minutes on each side, or until lightly and evenly browned. Remove the veal from the pan, set aside and keep warm.

Add the bacon to the pan and cook, stirring constantly, for 1 minute. Stir in the tomato juice. Reduce the heat to low and simmer for 5 minutes.

Stir in the capers and add the wine. Bring the mixture to the boil, stirring frequently. Pour the sauce over the veal and serve immediately.

Chicken Livers with Mushrooms
SERVES 1

1 teaspoon vegetable oil
2 large chicken livers, diced
1 tablespoon chopped onion
1 tablespoon chopped, fresh parsley
4 large mushrooms, with stalks reserved and chopped
1 tablespoon cottage cheese
½ teaspoon lemon juice
½ teaspoon garlic powder
2 tablespoons hot chicken stock (optional)

Preheat the oven to 180°C (350°F), gas mark 4.

Heat the oil in a frying-pan. Add the livers and cook, stirring constantly, for 2 minutes. Add the onion and parsley and cook, stirring frequently, for 3 minutes. Add the mushroom stalks and cook, stirring occasionally, for 5 minutes.

Remove the pan from the heat and stir in the cottage cheese. Set aside and keep warm.

Arrange the mushroom caps, the smooth side downwards, in a shallow, ovenproof dish. Spoon the liver mixture into the mushroom caps and sprinkle over the lemon juice. Cover with foil and bake for 30 minutes.

Sprinkle over a little garlic powder just before serving and add the chicken stock, if desired.

Seafood Special
SERVES 1

1 teaspoon vegetable oil
1 tablespoon chopped onion
1 garlic clove, crushed
½ tomato, chopped
⅛ teaspoon saffron
225 g (8 oz) mixed seafood (prawns, shrimps, mussels, cockles, oysters)
1 slice High Protein Bread, toasted and cut into triangles
1 tablespoon chopped, fresh parsley

Heat the oil in a frying-pan. Add the onion, garlic and tomato and cook, stirring occasionally, for 5 minutes.

Add the saffron and mixed seafood and cook, stirring frequently, for 2 minutes. Cover and bring to the boil.

Transfer the mixture to a serving plate and garnish with the toast triangles. Sprinkle over the parsley and serve immediately.

Lamb, Greek-style
SERVES 1

125-225 g (4-8 oz) lamb fillet
½ teaspoon vegetable oil
4 tablespoons cooked rice
1 tablespoon chopped onion
salt and pepper
4 vine leaves, blanched
50 ml (2 fl oz) chicken stock

Preheat the oven to 180°C (350°F), gas mark 4. Brush the lamb on both sides with the oil.

Roast the lamb, turning once, for 25-30 minutes, or until it is cooked through and tender.

Meanwhile, mix together the rice and onion and add salt and pepper to taste. Place one-quarter of the mixture on each vine leaf. Roll up the leaves, tucking in the sides, to form parcels.

Place the vine leaf parcels, seam side downwards, in a shallow, ovenproof dish. Pour over the chicken stock. Place in the oven and cook for 20 minutes.

Serve the lamb with the vine leaf parcels.

Fish Tabasco
SERVES 1

125 g (4 oz) fresh, filleted salmon, mackerel or
*   halibut*
2 tablespoons chopped onion
1 tablespoon chopped chives
¼ teaspoon tabasco sauce
50 ml (2 fl oz) lemon juice
1 large tomato, chopped
2 lemon wedges

Preheat the oven to 180°C (350°F), gas mark 4. Cut out a large square of foil.

Place the fish on the foil and bring up the sides to form a container. Sprinkle the onion, chives, tabasco sauce and lemon juice over the fish. Fold over the foil, tucking in the sides, to form a secure parcel. Bake for 25 minutes.

Unseal the foil and add the tomato. Reseal the foil and cook for a further 5 minutes.

Transfer the fish to a serving plate, garnish with the lemon wedges and serve immediately.

Chicken and Seafood Sauté
SERVES 1

1 chicken breast
175 ml (6 fl oz) water
1 teaspoon vegetable oil
50 g (2 oz) shrimps, shelled
50 g (2 oz) frozen peas
4 canned asparagus spears, drained
50 g (2 oz) mushrooms, sliced
25 g (1 oz) blanched almonds

Put the chicken breast in a small saucepan and pour over the water. Bring to the boil, reduce the heat to low and simmer for 6 minutes.

Meanwhile, heat the oil in a frying-pan. Add the shrimps and cook, stirring frequently, for 5 minutes, or until they turn pink in colour.

Remove the shrimps from the pan, set aside and keep warm.

Add the peas to the pan and cook, stirring frequently, for 1 minute. Add the asparagus spears and heat gently until they are warmed through.

Add the mushrooms to the saucepan with the chicken and cook for a further 3 minutes.

Transfer the chicken and mushrooms to a warm serving plate. Surround with the shrimps, peas and asparagus and garnish with almonds.

Desserts

Desserts suitable for Keep Trim meals are zero-carbohydrate jellies, glacées and moulds and low calorie fruits seasoned with lemon or ginger. Traditional recipes which do not contain flour or sugar are also permitted.

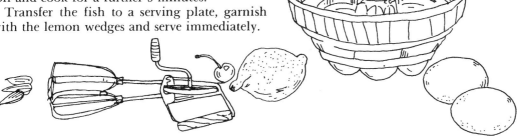

What next?

It may come as a shock to the gourmet eater that he must now go back on the SMD for a further two weeks. However, what can be expected from the dedicated adherent to the Scarsdale Plan can be seen from the graph.

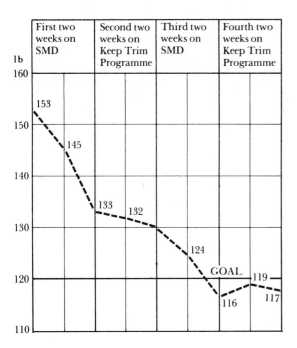

Once you have reached your desired weight then you must follow the Keep Trim routine for evermore. Every Scarsdale dieter is enjoined to weigh himself weekly. A 1.8 kg (4 lb) increase over your desired weight is an instant direction to go back on the SMD for a further two weeks. How many succeed in Dr Tarnower's proud claim to lose up to 9 kg (20 lb) in 14 days? The answer remains somewhat problematical. Based on the Keep Trim routine Dr Tarnower developed a weight maintenance programme which he called 'How to be a lifetime winner'. This is discussed in Chapter XIV.

The Pritikin Diet

Almost as if to prove that there is a diet that suits everyone, the Pritikin Diet (named after its inventor Nathan Pritikin) has recently been developed. In a way, it is *the diet* for the vegetarian, who finds dieting extremely difficult, and for the person who likes carbohydrate too much to face a day without it. It is designed as a high carbohydrate, low protein, very low fat diet, but it is also something else (almost by accident). It includes high quantities of vegetable fibre.

Just in case this looks like an ideal diet for those whose idea of good food is massive sugary pastries and a free run of the confectionery department, let me define a little more closely what Nathan Pritikin means by carbohydrate. Like all good diet experts he abhors the empty (simple) carbohydrate calorie—sugar, molasses, syrup. His carbohydrate is fibre-rich (complex) carbohydrate—whole grain cereal and vegetables. (High fibre foods are also discussed in Chapter XIV.) There is good evidence to suggest that fibre-depleted diets are related to a high incidence of diverticulitis, piles, varicose veins, hiatus hernia, gallstones, large bowel cancer and perhaps appendicitis. High fibre in the diet is associated with a low incidence of coronary and other arterial diseases. It is an interesting fact that if you design a high fibre-high carbohydrate diet it also turns out to be a low fat diet, mainly to save on calories. Now *if* low fat diets *are* a major factor in reducing 'clotability' factors in the blood, then of course such diets are moving all the time in the direction of reducing cardiovascular diseases.

Actually, the Pritikin Diet is (like all successful diets) more than a diet. It includes an increased exercise quotient as part and parcel of its package deal. Exercise not only helps you to lose weight, it also protects you against cardiovascular disease. It does this in two ways. First, it lessens the hazard of 'high clotability' in the blood and, second, it increases 'exercise tolerance'. Some people, if they happen to be of an athletic turn of mind, talk about 'training'. Training means getting the body used to increased periods of activity. As a result, you can walk up hills and climb stairs very much more easily without getting 'puffed out' or short of breath.

There is an interesting corollary involving a very specialized type of training. You can get 'in training' for a heart attack. Or more directly, in training to survive a heart attack. Far too many heart attacks are fatal and kill within minutes. The heart is a simple muscular pump. Like all pumps it needs power to keep going. The unfit heart with little reserve power developed by exercise (training) sometimes has so little in reserve that it immediately fails if one tiny area of its muscle power is knocked out by a sudden heart attack. A fine robust heart can often keep going even if five or ten times such an area is suddenly affected by a heart attack.

Naturally, therefore, a diet which has so much going for it in terms of disease prevention is a good diet. Thus the success of the Pritikin Diet. In the United States, from where this diet hails, the Pritikin Diet is linked strongly with a behavioural type of eating modification regime (see Chapter VII). There is a Longevity Centre at Santa Barbara in California where patients enrol for a four-week programme of low-calorie meals (unlimited in quantity, eight meals a day) and exercise. It is claimed that they lose over 6 kg (13 lb) during four weeks on this regime. Community-based Pritikin Better Health Programmes also operate in the United States.

Certain foods, many of which most of us would consider aids to civilized living, are forbidden on the Pritikin regime and these include eggs, natural milk, cheese, butter, margarine, soya bean products. Oils are also prohibited, together with sugars and alcohol. Only modest quantities of protein are allowed per day—100 g (3½ oz) of lean meat, poultry and fish, 1 egg white, 225 ml (8 fl oz) skimmed milk. High protein vegetables (beans and peas) are allowed in 100 g (3½ oz) portions with the meat or fish course. All other vegetables, grains (whole rice, barley and wheat) and wholemeal grain products are allowed in unlimited quantities. 25 g (1 oz) of gelatine is allowed per week.

It has been suggested that the successful Pritikin Diet is a puritan or a masochistic diet—or both. Food additives are studiously avoided, and so are tea, coffee and alcohol. There is a pre-occupation with natural foods.

Not permitted foods

Fats
Oils
Sugars
Fat meat
Offal
Milk (except skimmed milk)
Egg yolks
Cheeses (except less than 1 per cent fat by weight)
Nuts (except chestnuts)
Seeds (except grains)
Soya beans
Avocados
Olives
Cooked, canned or frozen fruit with sugar
Jam
Syrup
Grain products made with added fats or egg yolks (some pastas)
Salt in excess of 4 g per day
Mayonnaise
Sandwich spreads
Gravies
Sauces
Most dessert items (containing fats, oils, sugars, egg yolks)
Sweets, chocolate and other confectionery
Alcoholic drinks (small quantity light white wine allowed)
Tea
Coffee
Cola drinks

Sample menu

A day on a Pritikin regime might include the following:

BREAKFAST
Half a grapefruit
Bowl of cooked whole-grain cereal with fruit, skimmed milk and bran

LUNCH
Bowl of vegetable soup
Large wholemeal bumper sandwich containing green salad, pickled vegetables, sprinkled with vinegar, lemon and bran

DINNER
Meat soup
Steamed broccoli
Courgettes
Brown rice
Salad
Wholemeal bread
Stewed apples
Yogurt

SNACKS
Three snacks of either fruit, salad or wholemeal sandwiches

The 'Free' Diet

This diet is suitable for people who can make a package deal with themselves to eat certain foods and avoid others. It has also proved successful with slimming groups. The diet contains no sugar, is low in starch, moderate in fat content and high in protein. It is known as a 'free' diet because the slimmer is allowed unrestricted quantities of a wide range of enjoyable foods, but, at the same time, all other foods are given up entirely. Weight-loss will be between 500 g and 1.75 kg (1-4 lb) per week

General rules

1 **Eat as much of the permitted foods as you like.**
2 **Do not eat any other foods, particularly foods containing refined sugar or flour.**
3 **Eat three or four meals a day.**
4 **Do not eat between meals.**
5 **You are allowed 275 ml (½ pint) milk per day, including milk taken in coffee and tea.**
6 **You are allowed 25 g (1 oz) butter, margarine or cream per day.**
7 **You are allowed one or two potatoes per day.**
8 **You are allowed 75 g (3 oz) starch-reduced bread, six pieces of crispbread or six starch-reduced rolls per day. Instead of 25 g (1 oz) bread you may have EITHER a small helping of plain cereal or pasta OR 275 ml (½ pint) beer OR one glass of spirits OR 25 g (1 oz) sweets.**
9 **To make the diet more effective, omit peas, beans (except runner), parsnips, sweetcorn and grapes.**
10 **If you cannot keep to low carbohydrate foods, limit your cheese intake to 50 g (2 oz) per day.**
11 **If you suffer from constipation, take up to 25 g (1 oz) bran daily.**

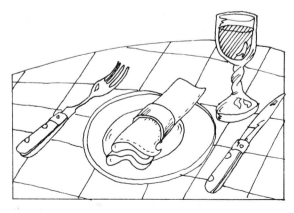

Permitted foods

Lean meat
Poultry
Liver
Kidneys
Lean ham
Bacon
Grilled sausages
Fish
Eggs
Cheese
Cottage cheese
Salads
Vegetables
Fresh fruit (except bananas)
Fruit bottled without sugar
Nuts (as part of a main dish)
Consomme
Sour pickles
Thin soups
Worcestershire sauce
Tea
Coffee
Low-calorie drinks

Not permitted

All foods not listed above, including all foods containing refined sugar and flour

Bread (except daily allowance)
Biscuits
Cake
Pastry
Cereals (except daily allowance)
Dried or canned fruit
Butter or margarine (except daily allowance)
Cream (except daily allowance)
Milk (except daily allowance)
Thick sauces
Thick soups
Puddings
Ice-cream
Sugar
Syrup
Chocolate
Sweets
Cocoa
Honey
Jam
Alcohol (except daily allowance)
Sweetened fruit drinks
Tonic water

Low Fat Diet

Low fat dieting is popular because many people are rather frightened of fat as an element of nutrition—whether or not you should be frightened of fat is, of course, debatable. Low fat diets do have certain advantages. Weight for weight, fat is very calorific and therefore by excluding fat from your diet you can eat larger quantities of other foods and reduce the number of calories to a level at which weight-loss will occur.

There is the equivalent of 3,500 calories in 500 g (1 lb) of body fat. To lose weight you need to reduce calorie intake so that the body can use stored fat in the fat cells for energy. If you normally eat 2,000 calories a day and you reduce this by 500, you will lose about 500 g (1 lb) of actual fat a week. During the first week you will also lose water, making the weight-loss appear greater.

Fats have an energy-providing function, they help in transporting fat-soluble vitamins around the body, are necessary for healthy skin and, as they are slow to digest, they satisfy hunger. We normally eat more than 40 per cent of our daily calories as fat, visible or invisible in foods, and this figure is considered by doctors to be too high.

Experts consider that too much *saturated* fat (animal fats such as butter, lard, full-fat milk, hard cheese, margarine, fatty meats and coconut oil) helps to raise blood cholesterol and this *may* contribute to the risks of coronary heart disease. However, polyunsaturated fat (in soft margarines, sunflower and corn oil) actually reduces cholesterol levels.

Obesity and a high consumption of fat in the normal diet seem to go together. In countries such as Korea (where each person eats eight per cent of fat per day) and in Japan, there is not as much obesity as there is in the West. Rationing fats is a good way to cut calories.

General Rules

1 Do not eat foods with a high fat content.
2 You may eat plenty of vegetables, and also cereals and sugar-free carbohydrates such as potatoes, pasta, rice and bread.
3 Drink skimmed milk.
4 Eat more vegetable-based dishes, avoiding dishes with meat as the main ingredient.
5 Avoid cakes, pastry, biscuits, and made-up desserts which are high in sugar as well as fats.
6 Do not eat fried foods.

Foods with a very high fat content

Fried foods
Lard
Butter
Vegetable oil
Olive oil
Margarine
Avocado pear
Bacon
Peanuts
Brazil nuts
Walnuts
Pork chops
Pork sausages
Salami
Pastry
Mayonnaise
Salad cream
Biscuits
Coconut
Potato crisps
Chips
Hard cheeses
Cream cheese
Suet
Dripping
Cakes
Fatty meats
Cream
Chocolate

Foods with a fairly high fat content

Eggs
Tuna fish
Curd cheese
Camembert
Edam
Cocoa
Corned beef
Cooked ham
Stewed beef
Beef sausages
Cheese spread
Ice-cream
Herrings
Kippers
Sardines
Lean roast beef
Lean roast lamb
Croissants
Kedgeree
Baked egg custard

Low fat slimming meals

Sample menus are given for two weeks of low fat dieting. They are based on 1,000 calories per day and contain enough protein, vitamins, minerals and fibre to keep you in good health. The fat content accounts for about one third of the daily energy intake, and this is much lower than normal. Your daily allowance of milk is 275 ml (½ pint). Avoid alcohol when following this diet.

WEEK 1	MONDAY	TUESDAY	WEDNESDAY
BREAKFAST	4 tablespoons cornflakes 125 (5 fl oz) skimmed milk 1 teaspoon sugar	2 slices wholemeal toast spread thinly with low fat spread 2 teaspoons marmalade	200 ml (7 fl oz) porridge 1 teaspoon sugar
LUNCH	5 tablespoons lean beef stew Medium-sized baked potato 2 tablespoons peas	Pasta salad made with 75 g (3 oz) pasta shells, 50 g (2 oz) chopped lean, cooked meat, 1 apple, lettuce, 1 tablespoon low-calorie dressing	200 g (7 oz) cod steaks, poached Grilled tomatoes 1 slice wholemeal bread spread thinly with low fat spread 1 apple
DINNER	200 g (7 oz) plaice fillet, brushed with 2 teaspoons melted butter before grilling Small bunch grapes Whole French beans 2 tablespoons mousse	175 g (6 oz) roast pork fillet stuffed with prunes 4 tablespoons spinach with nutmeg 1 tablespoon sour cream 4 tablespoons fresh fruit salad	6 tablespoons chilli con carne 3 tablespoons carrots 1 medium-sized boiled potato

WEEK 2	MONDAY	TUESDAY	WEDNESDAY
BREAKFAST	3 tablespoons bran 140 g (5 fl oz) carton plain yogurt	1 orange 1 slice wholemeal toast spread thinly with low fat spread 1 teaspoon marmalade	2 rashers well-grilled bacon Grilled tomatoes
LUNCH	Chicken Waldorf salad, made with 50 g (2 oz) cooked, diced chicken, ½ diced apple, ½ tablespoon walnuts, 1 tablespoon raisins, 2 tablespoons cooked peas, 1 tablespoon low-calorie dressing	3 grilled fish fingers 1 tablespoon low-calorie tartare sauce Sliced green beans 1 slice wholemeal bread	Toasted sandwich, made with 2 slices bread spread with mustard or cranberry jelly, 50 g (2 oz) lean cooked lamb, 50 g (2 oz) cottage cheese, lettuce and cucumber
DINNER	5 tablespoons sweet and sour pork (using lean pork) 150 g (5 oz) noodles Bean sprouts	5 tablespoons beef stew 3 tablespoons potato mashed with skimmed milk Braised green cabbage Peach, fresh or baked	Paella, made with 125 g (4 oz) cooked rice, 50 g (2 oz) each of cooked chicken, cod, mussels, prawns, 2 tablespoons peas 1 fresh or canned pear

THURSDAY	FRIDAY	SATURDAY	SUNDAY
2 rashers well-grilled bacon 1 slice wholemeal bread	1 boiled egg 2 crispbreads spread thinly with low fat spread	4 tablespoons bran 175 ml (6 fl oz) skimmed milk 1 tablespoon raisins	140 g (5 fl oz) carton plain yogurt 1 small grapefruit 1 teaspoon sugar
Cottage cheese salad, made with 140 g (5 oz) cottage cheese, lettuce, tomato, watercress and orange 1 crispbread	2 stuffed tomatoes, filled with 1 sardine mashed with 2 tablespoons wholemeal breadcrumbs, lemon juice, 1 tablespoon plain yogurt	Open sandwich, made with wholemeal bread, spread with low-calorie salad dressing, 2 tablespoons prawns, 1 hard-boiled egg and salad	1 large baked potato, filled with 50 g (2 oz) chopped corned beef and chutney
75 g (3 oz) liver baked in foil with onion and mushrooms Courgettes baked and tossed in 2 tablespoons plain yogurt 4 tablespoons brown rice 4 tablespoons stewed fruit 2 tablespoons single cream	2 slices lean lamb 2 small boiled potatoes Broccoli 2 tablespoons sweetcorn Banana, fresh or baked	Spaghetti Bolognese, made with 175 g (6 oz) cooked spaghetti, 4 tablespoons of meat sauce, 1 tablespoon Parmesan cheese	3 lambs' kidneys cooked in wine 4 tablespoons rice Baked courgettes and aubergines 1 glass of red or dry white wine

THURSDAY	FRIDAY	SATURDAY	SUNDAY
6 prunes 4 dried apricot halves, soaked and cooked 2 tablespoons bran 125 ml (5 fl oz) skimmed milk	150 ml (6 fl oz) porridge 1 tablespoon raisins	4 tablespoons cornflakes 1 sliced banana 125 ml (5 fl oz) skimmed milk	1 slice bread 1 rasher well-grilled bacon Poached mushrooms
Eggs Florentine, made with 2 poached eggs, 125 g (4 oz) cooked spaghetti and 175 g (6 oz) cooked spinach	Kedgeree, made with 4 tablespoons cooked rice, 75 g (3 oz) cooked smoked haddock, 6 g (¼ oz) butter and onion	Open sandwich, made with 1 slice rye bread spread with horseradish sauce, sliced cucumber, 1 slice lean roast beef and lettuce	1 hard-boiled egg 4 tablespoons cooked noodles in curry sauce 4 tablespoons fresh fruit salad
250 g (9 oz) chicken joint with skin removed, brushed with Worcestershire sauce and grilled 3 tablespoons sweetcorn and peppers 1 ring of pineapple Cauliflower	2 beef olives, made with beef, filled with breadcrumbs, beaten egg, anchovies and capers Broccoli or leeks 1 medium-sized baked potato Small portion mousse	175 g (6 oz) lean pork chop 4 tablespoons ratatouille made without fat 3 tablespoons potato Anna (thick layers of onion and potato baked in milk) 125 g (4 oz) fruit in meringue basket	2 ham and spinach pancakes Tomato sauce Mixed vegetables

(Courtesy of *Woman* magazine)

Foods with a low fat content

White fish
Poultry
Game
Kidneys
Liver
Rabbit
Tripe
Veal
Shellfish
Cottage cheese
Baked beans
Lentils
Barley
Oatmeal
Haricot beans
Vegetables
Fruit
Skimmed milk
Yogurt
Bread
Rice
Spaghetti
Pasta

The strange tale of Mr Banting

This is the oldest diet in the world which is known to have worked in practice. It also gives every failed dieter a two-fold cheering message. First, you are never too old to diet successfully and so extend your lifespan. Second, you do not have to live miserably to do it. Mr Banting gave us the word *to bant*—a verb which crept into the English language during the nineteenth century but which is now largely forgotten. He might, therefore, be described, as Mr Diet.

Mr Banting was a successful and prosperous London undertaker. Always a portly man, he reached a stage of advanced obesity, at the age of 66. He was only about 1.7 m (5 ft 5 in) tall and weighed 92 kg (202 lb). With even the most generous projections, his life expectancy at this stage of overweight presented a grim picture. It is not known whether or not he was alarmed at the prospect of his early demise, but we do know that one thing did depress him. He was so grossly obese that he could only negotiate stairs with extreme difficulty and this created serious problems in carrying out his profession. Furthermore, he was having difficulty in dressing himself. Naturally, he was driven into the arms of the medical profession, who advised first one treatment and then another, but, unfortunately, nothing helped. Some of the diets he was advised to follow made him get even fatter.

At this point, the story takes a mysterious turn. Mr Banting was becoming very deaf as well as very fat. He consulted an ear surgeon who incidentally persuaded Mr Banting to try a diet that he had developed. Mr Banting did so and was overjoyed. In less than a year he had lost about 23 kg (50 lb) and his waistline was reduced by a little over 30 cm (12 in). Oddly enough, fame did not fall to the ear surgeon, a Mr William Harvey, but to the fat undertaker himself, who published his gospel in 1864, two years after he himself had embarked on it.

Mr Banting's original diet

Breakfast   Up to 150 g (5 oz) of beef, mutton, kidneys, fish, bacon or any cold meats, except pork, were permitted. (This prohibition may have been due to the fact that, at this time, pork was often infested with worms rather than for any other dietary reason.) A biscuit, probably a home-baked water biscuit), or 25 g (1 oz) of dry toast was allowed and a cup of tea without milk or sugar.

Lunch The diet allowed up to 175 g (6 oz) of fish. (Banting stipulated 'except salmon', possibly because, in his day, it was thought a somewhat disreputable 'coarse' fish, rather than for any real dietary reason. Salmon is, as it happens, a fairly fatty fish very closely resembling fresh herring from the dieter's point of view.) 175 g (6 oz) of meat (again, excepting pork), poultry or game could be eaten as an alternative to fish. All vegetables, except potatoes, were allowed. Fruit provided the dessert. In addition, the dieter could have 25 g (1 oz) of dry toast and up to three glasses of 'good claret', sherry or Madeira. Under no circumstances, were champagne, port or beer allowed!

Tea This comprised up to 75 g (3 oz) of fruit, 'a rusk or two' and tea without milk or sugar.

Supper This consisted of the same choice as for lunch, but only two glasses of claret were allowed.

'Nightcap' If required, the dieter could take a glass or two of claret or sherry or a 'tumbler of grog' (gin, whisky or brandy with water).

Does it work?

It is difficult to calculate the calorie content of such a diet, but it would probably amount to around 3,000 per day. In effect, it was a high fat, high protein, low carbohydrate diet, which permitted a considerable alcohol content.

Does the Banting diet work? It certainly did for Banting as the following analysis shows:

August 1862	92 kg	(202 lb)
Christmas 1862	83 kg	(184 lb)
August 1863	71 kg	(156 lb)

Clearly for fat people, the carbohydrates are the culprits. Also, the dictum that carbohydrates = alcohol, on this score, does not always hold good.

Bogus diets

If a diet sounds too wonderful or seems to be sold too hard, then think about it very carefully. For example, at some time almost every fruit under the sun has been hailed as the greatest natural diet ever and enthusiastic devotees have sat down to weeks on nothing but oranges, grapefruit or bananas. Some years ago raw fruit and raw vegetables formed the basis of fashionable slimming diets. There is only one thing wrong with such diets. If they contain fewer calories than the slimmer needs, weight is certainly lost, but, as such diets do not contain enough protein, the slimmer breaks up his own muscle and subsequently starts to lose weight very rapidly. Muscular weakness and spinal pains soon supervene, as malnutrition sets in with a vengeance. When you hear of such diets, think twice or even three times.

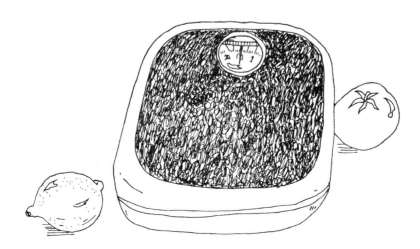

CHAPTER IX

Diet wreckers

Alcohol and fast foods can play havoc with a dietary regime. It is wise to restrict alcohol intake to one glass of dry white wine a day and to avoid all high-calorie foods.

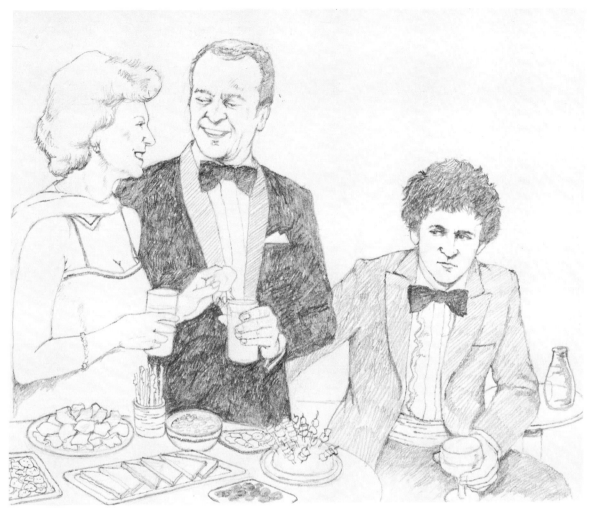

Many doctors and dieticians have been ambiguous about alcohol and slimming. One diet book even says that alcohol contains no carbohydrate, while its mere chemical formula, C_2H_5OH, labels it a mixture of carbon, hydrogen and oxygen. To be completely fair, it must be said that it is not a carbohydrate in the strictly technical sense, simply because of the way the elements are joined to each other. Nevertheless, the body makes no such technical distinctions in its treatment of alcohol as a carbohydrate.

In fact, alcohol occupies a rather special place as far as weight-gain is concerned. One slimming expert says, 'If someone on a diet must have alcohol, let him get drunk once a week.' This will certainly not do his liver much good, but in another way, the advice is sound.

If you drink an entire bottle of whisky in one night, then, as the blood alcohol rapidly rises, the body 'loses' more and more alcohol into the urine and in the breath. Unless the body could get rid of alcohol in this way, quite a small quantity of spirits would kill rapidly. Similarly, the liver 'burns up' and 'detoxifies' alcohol at an increased rate too. In other words, high blood alcohol equals rapid alcohol loss. However, if you divide your bottle of whisky (or gin, rum or brandy) into seven portions and take these every night, this rapid loss of alcohol does not happen. Instead the body tends to treat alcohol like a surplus carbohydrate. In other words, it treats alcohol as a food. Consequently, you have to add alcoholic drinks to your calorie list if you are a slimmer. You are certainly not recommended to get blind drunk one night of the week.

Another problem with alcoholic drinks is that they stimulate the appetite, hence the traditional glass of sherry before dinner. Moreover, except, perhaps, for large quantities of weak beer, alcohol has no satiety value, unless you drink a vast and intoxicating amount. Alcohol, therefore, encourages food intake.

Finally, and this is where many diets falter, some alcoholic drinks contain sugar in addition to alcohol.

Liqueurs are perhaps the easiest of all drinks to refuse and to avoid. This is just as well for slimmers, as they are all highly calorific. Also, remember that what you mix with your drink can make a tremendous difference from the slimming point of view.

A good working rule for alcohol and slimming is as follows. You may have one drink a day (particularly older adults), if you allow for the calories supplied by the drink and omit an appropriate and corresponding amount of other food. No snacks, such as peanuts or crisps, are permitted, unless you count those calories too.

The drinker's diet

It is accepted that alcohol plays a special part in the genesis of obesity. However, alcohol plays such a large part in many people's lives that

Beer drinkers' guide

BEER	ALCOHOL g PER 570 ml (1 pint)	CALORIES PER 570 ml (1 pint)
Bitter (draught)	17.4	177
Brown ale (bottled)	12.7	159
Mild (draught)	14.8	144
Pale ale (bottled)	19.0	184
Stout (bottled)	16.3	212
Stout (extra)	24.2	223
Strong ale	37.7	414

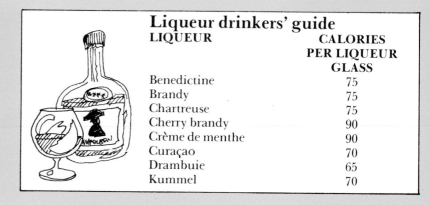

Liqueur drinkers' guide

LIQUEUR	CALORIES PER LIQUEUR GLASS
Benedictine	75
Brandy	75
Chartreuse	75
Cherry brandy	90
Crème de menthe	90
Curaçao	70
Drambuie	65
Kummel	70

Soft drinks and mixers guide

SOFT DRINK	CALORIES PER 100 ml	CALORIES PER fl oz
American ginger ale	39	11
Bitter lemon	32	9
Cola drink	41	12
Dry ginger ale	14	4
Ginger beer	39	11
Glucose drink	75	21
Soda water	0	0
Tonic water	21	6

simply to eliminate it from their diets and to change their eating habits at the same time is usually too much for regular drinkers to contemplate. This problem led to the concept of a Drinking Man's Diet. There is no magic in this. First, the drinker decides how much he wants to drink each day, he then adds up the number of alcohol calories and subtracts them from his carbohydrate calorie allowance.

There are many built-in snags to any drinker's diet. Often the substitutions make what is left of the diet unpalatable and unsatisfactory, and it is therefore soon abandoned. Another disadvantage is that alcohol is a great postponer of decisions, especially difficult decisions, and so the 'just this once I'll have some chips' factor creeps in and any idea of consistent dieting goes by the board. Perhaps the most difficult factor with reference to drink and food is that the former gives us an appetite to enjoy the latter—usually much more of the latter. By and large, a drinker's diet does not work. If the drinker is intent on losing weight, then it is far better for him to impose a strict limit on the drink that is allowed within his chosen diet (e.g. a glass of white wine) and to confine the rest of his drinking to zero-calorie tonics and sodas.

Wine drinkers' guide

WINE	ALCOHOL PER CENT	CALORIES PER 100 ml (3½ fl oz)
Claret	9.68	69
Champagne (dry)	10.95	83
Champagne (sweet)	8.49	80
Graves	9.80	70
Greek wine	12.35	87
Hock	9.73	68
Hungarian wine	10.16	71
Madeira	17.82	132
Marsala	16.80	130
Moselle	8.54	60
Port	18.11	136
Sauterne	10.22	73
Sauterne (sweet)	9.34	71
Sherry	17.80	136

Cider drinkers' guide

CIDER	ALCOHOL g PER 570 ml (1 pint)	CALORIES PER 570 ml (1 pint)
Dry cider	21.5	209
Sweet cider	20.9	158
Vintage cider	59.4	577

Spirits drinkers' guide

SPIRIT	QUANTITY	CALORIES
Bourbon	42 ml (1½ fl oz)	105
Brandy	30 ml (1 fl oz)	75
Gin	42 ml (1½ fl oz)	105
Rum	42 ml (1½ fl oz)	105
Rye whiskey	42 ml (1½ fl oz)	105
Scotch whisky	42 ml (1½ fl oz)	105
Vodka	42 ml (1½ fl oz)	105

Banned and substitute foods

It can be quite a problem 'sticking' to your diet, especially when it comes to ordering food in a restaurant or preparing meals for other people as well as for yourself. Do not let other people dictate what you can eat, but be very strict with yourself. The following lists of forbidden foods and of substitutes are a life-line for the dieter who is almost 'on the rocks'.

INSTEAD OF:	Calories	SUBSTITUTE:	Calories
DRINKS			
Beer (1 bottle)	175	42 ml (1½ fl oz) spirits with soda water or water	105
225 ml (8 fl oz) chocolate milk shake	500	225 ml (8 fl oz) lemonade	90
225 ml (8 fl oz) cocoa (all milk)	235	225 ml (8 fl oz) cocoa (milk and water)	140
Coffee with cream and 2 teaspoons sugar	110	Black coffee with artificial sweetener	0
110 ml (4 fl oz) orange juice	50	1 cup consomme	10
225 ml (8 fl oz) soft drinks	90	225 ml (8 fl oz) diet soft drinks	1 or 2
BREAKFAST			
Even small modifications in the way eggs are cooked can lead to considerable calorie savings.			
2 eggs, scrambled	240	2 eggs, boiled or poached	160
1-1½ cups cornflakes or bran	110	1 cup puffed rice or puffed wheat	50
DAIRY PRODUCTS			
You can tell that margarine is better than butter when it comes to economizing on calories.			
2 pats of butter	100	2 pats of low-calorie margarine	34
25 g (1 oz) blue, Cheddar, cream or Emmenthal cheese	100	25 g (1 oz) cottage cheese	25
CAKES			
Perhaps exchanging a slice of melon for your favourite angel cake may seem hard, but the calorie savings are considerable.			
5 cm (2 in) slice angel cake	110	Slice water melon	40
5 cm (2 in) slice cheesecake	200	Slice melon	60
5 cm (2 in) slice iced chocolate cake	525	5 cm (2 in) slice sponge cake	120
Iced cupcake	230	Plain cupcake	115
5 cm (2 in) slice fruit cake	115	1 cup of grapes	65

INSTEAD OF:	Calories	SUBSTITUTE:	Calories

DESSERTS

Clearly, choosing your desserts from the fresh fruit counter is better than going for pies and tarts.

INSTEAD OF:	Calories	SUBSTITUTE:	Calories
1 piece apple pie	338	1 small orange	40-50
1 piece custard tart	280	1 small banana	85
110 ml (4 fl oz) ice-cream	150	110 ml (4 fl oz) flavoured yogurt	60
1 piece lemon meringue pie	305	½ cup flavoured jelly	70

MEAT AND FISH

The different cuts of meat do have a considerable bearing on the calorie content. Choose fish carefully too.

INSTEAD OF:	Calories	SUBSTITUTE:	Calories
75 g (3 oz) canned tuna	165	75 g (3 oz) canned crabmeat	80
75 g (3 oz) grilled hamburger (average fat)	240	75 g (3 oz) grilled hamburger (lean)	145
75 g (3 oz) lamb chop	300	75 g (3 oz) roast leg of lamb (lean only)	160
Meat loaf	680	Rump steak	320
75 g (3 oz) pork sausage	405	75 g (3 oz) boiled ham (lean)	200
75 g (3 oz) Porterhouse steak	250	75 g (3 oz) rump steak	160
75 g (3 oz) roast duck	310	75 g (3 oz) roast chicken	160
75 g (3 oz) roast pork	310	75 g (3 oz) roast veal	230
75 g (3 oz) roast topside of beef	290	75 g (3 oz) roast rib of beef	220

SANDWICHES

A bumper sandwich can be very high in calories compared with an egg salad sandwich.

INSTEAD OF:	Calories	SUBSTITUTE:	Calories
Average sandwich	375	Bacon and tomato sandwich	200
Peanut butter sandwich	275	Egg salad sandwich	165

Banned and substitute foods (continued)

INSTEAD OF:	Calories	SUBSTITUTE:	Calories

SNACKS

Snacks are best avoided, but if your will is weak, grapes and pretzels score heavily over peanuts and chocolate.

INSTEAD OF:	Calories	SUBSTITUTE:	Calories
25 g (1 oz) chocolate	145	4 marshmallows (toasted)	80
1 cup shelled, roasted peanuts	1375	1 cup grapes	65
25 g (1 oz) salted peanuts	170	1 apple	80
10 medium-sized crisps	115	10 small pretzel sticks	35

SOUPS

Soups can be quite nourishing (calorific) but it is possible to economize greatly by sticking to clear soups.

1 cup vegetable soup	190	1 cup beef noodle soup	110
1 cup cream soup	210	1 cup chicken noodle soup	110
1 cup minestrone	105	1 cup beef bouillon	10

VEGETABLES

Vegetables are usually the dieter's friend —but beware of baked beans, sweetcorn and canned peas.

1 cup baked beans	320	1 cup green beans	30
1 cup sweetcorn	185	1 cup cauliflower	30
1 cup canned peas	145	12 asparagus spears	40

POTATOES

Usually, people equate slimming with not eating potatoes. In actual fact, it is possible to serve them in a relatively low-calorie form.

1 cup fried potatoes	480	6 cm (2½ in) baked potato	100
1 cup mashed potato	245	6 cm (2½ in) boiled potato	100

Note: 1 cup = 225 ml (8 fl oz)

Fast food equals fast fat

It seems that fast food for city dwellers is almost obligatory these days. If you have to eat a few fast food meals a week, it is best simply to log the calories, as the protein/fat/carbohydrate content is so variable. A calorie list of some fast food favourites is given.

Fast foods calorie counter

FISH	Calories
Fish, chips and coleslaw (large)	1100
Fish, chips and coleslaw (small)	905
McDonald's Filet-O-Fish	406

HAMBURGERS, ETC.	
Cheeseburger	305
Hamburger (according to size)	250-630
Double hamburger	350
Quarter pounder	414
Quarter pounder with cheese	521
Big Mac	557
Hot dog	291

CHICKEN	
Kentucky Fried Chicken	
Drumstick	220
Three piece special	660
Dinner (chicken, mashed potatoes, gravy, coleslaw, roll)	
2 piece Original	595
3 piece Original	830
2 piece Crispy	665
3 piece Crispy	1070
Half chicken (4 pieces)	625

CHIPS AND FRIES	Calories
French fries (average portion)	220
Onion rings	341

PIZZAS	
Individual 18 cm (7 in) pizza	1030
Half of 33 cm (13 in) pizza	900
Half of 38 cm (15 in) pizza	1200

DESSERTS	
Apple pie	265
Apple turnover	290
Banana split	580
Fruit sundae (small)	190
Fruit sundae (large)	430
Hot fudge sundae	580
Parfait	460

ICE-CREAM	
Ice-cream, plain cone	170

CAKES AND DOUGHNUTS	
Chocolate cake	250
Jam doughnut	275
Plain cake	240
Plain honey cake	260
Sugared doughnut	255
Add 50 calories for fillings	

SHAKES	
Fruit milk shake	320
Chocolate milk shake	365

CHAPTER X

The fat child

Children tend to be plump at certain ages and research is at present being carried out into whether adult obesity starts in childhood.

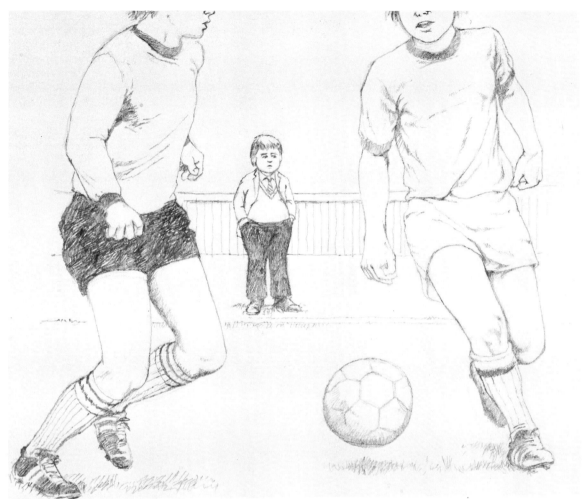

If someone is fat, was he born that way or is it the result of overeating or lack of exercise? There is quite a lot of evidence, at least, in animals, that genetic (inborn) tendencies are very closely related to body weight. Animal breeders can select 'strains' of pigs which fatten well, that is, without needing too much food. Beef cattle and sheep can be bred to produce a lot of lean meat. Happily perhaps, nobody has got around to breeding fatties and thinnies in the human race.

Twins and fatness

Much has been learned about human heredity and fatness from recent studies of pairs of twins. There are two types of twins. Identical twins come from a single fertilized egg which divides to form two more or less identical people. Fraternal twins come from two different egg cells which develop separately but simultaneously. These non-identi-cal twins are really just brothers and sisters of exactly the same age.

One of the reasons why it is so difficult to investigate the role of heredity in overweight people is that the ways in which different parents rear their children are so very variable. However, it is reasonable to assume that a pair of twins will be reared in more or less the same way by their parents. This is why studies of twins are of such interest to geneticists.

The weights of identical twins can be recorded at regular intervals. There will be some difference between them, but it will be very much less than the difference between non-identical twins. These inborn factors can be further studied in relation to body weight. For example, it is possible to record and study the weights of identical twins separated at birth and raised in different families. These twins will show greater variations in weight than identical twins raised in the same family.

Nevertheless, the variations will still be less than those between non-identical twins raised in similar circumstances. Thus the fine thread of nature and nurture runs through the whole fabric of fatness and thinness in childhood.

It can also be most informative to look closely at what happens to the children of overweight people as they grow up. If one parent is overweight, then 40-50 per cent of his or her children will be overweight when they grow up. If both parents are obese, the percentage increases to 70-80 per cent. It seems likely, therefore, that genetic factors are very important in determining eventual body weight.

Fat or plump?

Overweight children can be divided into two classes. The first and more unusual class might be called the 'hard cases'. These are the Billy and Bessie Bunters whom everybody finds so funny in fiction, but who are so tragic in fact. They are accused of being greedy, slothful, stupid and slow, but, in fact, they are blameless on this score. Some of these children have glandular problems, but most are perfectly healthy—and very fat. Their obesity is difficult to control with drugs, behavioural treatment or diets. Happily, most of them grow out of their fatness, but a few do not. Perhaps one day, medical science will find a way to help them. Until then, we should try to understand their humiliations and problems and avoid ridicule and rejection. The large majority of overweight children is outside this group. They are plump rather than fat.

Whether the seeds of adult obesity are sown in childhood is of great interest and a little more knowledge of this subject might well be a health investment for the future. Unfortunately too few facts are known, but those which are are highly interesting and our knowledge is expanding all the time.

The 'fat' organ

One way of looking at the problem of overweight is to view it as a disorder of a special organ—the *adipose* organ. Adipose tissue is connective tissue containing fat. In the same way as other organs in the body, such as the heart, are made of numerous individual cells, so the adipose organ has a cellular structure. This little piece of knowledge was seized with great enthusiasm a few years ago. It was suggested that how fat or thin you are depended upon how many adipose cells you had in your body and that, if you fattened up babies unduly, their fat cells increased in number and they would be fat for evermore. In fact, there has never been any convincing evidence that the number of fat cells an individual possesses makes the slightest difference to him. Fat cells seen under the microscope are all different sizes, but there are no giants. It seems likely that, as you get fat or thin, fat cells either duplicate themselves or shrivel down. So the 'fat for life' label on the overweight body has never been proved on the grounds of the cellular structure alone.

Critical Ages

It has been fairly clearly demonstrated that there are certain periods in a child's life when he tends to accumulate a lot of fat. These periods may be critical to what might be called subsequent 'fattability'.

The first of these critical periods is during the first nine months of life when the number of fat cells increases greatly. This is slightly more obvious in boys than in girls. After this quick 'fatten up' of infancy, fat is lost in both sexes until the ages of about eight to ten, although the *number* of fat cells does not decrease. Girls lose less fat than boys during these years.

An inference, which may be significant, can be drawn. The first nine months of life vary nutritionally from child to child, depending on one very simple factor—whether or not the mother breastfeeds her child. Breastfed children seldom become obese and the very common obesity of infancy is almost exclusively confined to the bottle-fed baby. At least one eminent nutritionist believes that an exaggeration of Nature's plumping up processes can carry the individual into later obesity.

The next obesity bonanza in children starts between the ages of 10 and 12 in boys and at puberty in girls, continuing into young womanhood. It seems likely that overnutrition at these critical periods has a lasting effect on the adipose organ. The theory postulates that, during these especially sensitive periods and primed by a multiplicity of factors, the adipose organ receives a lifelong 'message', dictating whether you will be a Mr Constant Weight or a Mrs Fatten Easily. Once these sensitive formative periods are over, the adipose organ becomes very resistant to change. Somehow, it has set its pattern. You *can* change it, as we have seen in earlier chapters, but there it will lie, waiting patiently for a calorie surplus, to dictate what your individual shape should be.

Nutritionists who subscribe to this theory believe that, if any great 'dent' is to be made in the vast epidemic of obesity bothering modern men and women, then careful monitoring of weight and dietary modification is essential during the times when the obesity organ is in its most sensitive state.

Fat babies

Although fatness in tiny babies can be measured by weighing them, another method provides a more accurate assessment. Special calipers are used to measure the thickness of 'skin-fold'. Previously, too much reliance on height and weight tables led to erroneous conclusions about overweight in children. A long baby will always appear 'overweight' when compared with a short one and will carry this degree of 'overweight' into childhood. However, this is not the same as being fat. Measures of skin-fold thickness have now been carried out for long enough for the difference between 'fatty' overweight and non-fatty overweight to be accurately assessed.

Fat children mature sooner

In girls, where body weight is closely related to the age at which menstruation starts, it is true that a fat child will mature earlier than her thin friend. The date of the menache is also related to the date at which the long bones (that give height) stop growing. Young girls who take the Pill for contraceptive purposes, or take Pill-like hormones for acne or painful periods, experience this hormone-stop in height in an exaggerated form and they are quite likely to become pocket-size Venuses. To some extent, the short adolescent turns into the over-fat adolescent.

High protein for children

The high protein form of dieting, described in Chapter VI, is particularly suitable for children and adolescents because their bodies need plenty of brick-building protein. The following table shows the effect of a high protein diet on a group of children who were all considerably overweight. Their ages ranged from 9 to 13 and they were each overweight by an average of 16 kg (36 lb). The rate of weight-loss slowed down over six months because children's bone content and the amount

of blood circulating increases all the time as they grow. On the very high protein diet, no bread or other carbohydrate food was allowed, but the diet was supplemented by the use of a dietetic loaf, rich in protein (25 per cent) and low in carbohydrate (16 per cent). On this diet, provided the dietary restrictions are maintained, all slimmers eventually revert to normal weight.

Months on diet	Diet*	Number on diet	Mean weight loss	% Success
1	MP	44	2.8	34
	VHP	41	4.7	64
4	MP	33	3.5	21
	VHP	36	8.7	50
6	MP	19	2.2	10
	VHP	16	8.0	40

* 1000 calories composed of:
MP (medium protein) = 40% protein, 20% fat, 40% carbohydrate
VHP (very high protein) = 57% protein, 26% fat, 17% carbohydrate

Guide for parents

Much obesity in the young is caused by the inactivity trap. Car travel, the school bus, constant excuses for not doing physical education at school, excessive television watching, TV meals, the lure of spectator rather than participant sports—all contribute to the under-exercised, overweight adolescent. Children will follow their parents' models in these matters. Diets should be worked out around a few rules.

1 **Give plenty of protein, particularly protein of animal origin such as fish and eggs.**
2 **Carbohydrates—anything goes except those foods rich in empty calories such as sugars, jam, honey, syrup, sweets, chocolates.**
3 **Limit milk to between 275-575 ml (½-1 pint) per day.**
4 **Hard foods that need chewing are better than soft foods.**
5 **The more food eaten, the more exercise needed.**
6 **Avoid alcoholic drinks.**
7 **Prepare meals that the rest of the family will enjoy too. Do not make the child feel excluded or uncomfortable.**
8 **Always emphasize what the overweight child may eat, rather than point out the foods that are forbidden.**
9 **Distract the child from food if possible.**

CHAPTER XI

Don't give up

There are many more failed dieters than successful ones. An understanding of diets and weight-loss helps the slimmer to shed those extra pounds for ever.

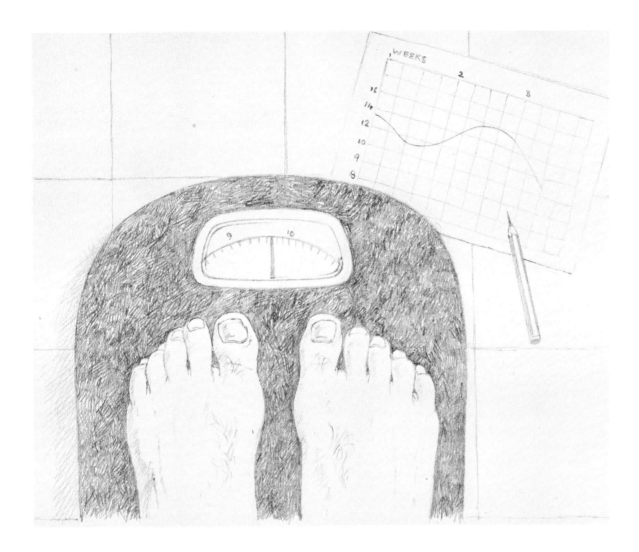

How many slimmers get fed up with their diets and give up, saying, 'After all, if the choice is fat and unfit or slim and miserable, why not stay overweight and be happy.'? Nobody actually knows the answer to this question, but probably the figure is quite high. There are certainly more failed dieters than successful ones and many more failures than are really necessary. There are innumerable reasons for failure, but it could often be prevented just by knowing a bit more about diets and weight-loss. The failures could so easily become success stories.

The failed dieter

One of the few well-documented analyses of failed dieters is that of the Department of Psychiatry at the University of Pennsylvania. Scientists looked at the effects of self-help groups for the treatment of obesity. They mainly studied a very popular group called TOPS (take off pounds sensibly), which had several thousand members, who were mostly white, almost exclusively female and usually in the 'pop' diet age bracket of 30-50. A typical member would be a 42-year-old woman. She would be some 58 per cent above her ideal weight and would lose about 6.8 kg (15 lb) during a membership of a little over 16 months.

TOPS offers a form of treatment similar to that of Weight Watchers, discussed in Chapter VII, involving group meetings and weigh-ins. It is therefore, a system about which the medical profession and nutritionists are currently expressing considerable enthusiasm. The loss of 6.8 kg

(15 lb) seems, at first sight, fairly good, but a closer look at **TOPS** shows that a high drop-out rate occurs. Fifty-four per cent of members 'survive' the first year and only 31 per cent are still members after two years. The prime cause for dropping out is failure to lose weight and dissatisfaction with the programme.

This is, of course, a comment on one isolated study and, apart from the studies mentioned in Chapter VII, we can hardly speak with scientific authority on what is the best slimming technique. In the heady world of diets and slimming, facts and figures are few and far between. However, 'blocks' to successful slimming seem to occur in all systems. Exactly how to solve the problems by effective trouble-shooting is, happily, gradually becoming better understood.

When and how to weigh

New slimmers are, naturally enough, obsessed with scales. Unfortunately, the scales often lie— and do so at times when, in fact, the slimmer is succeeding. If you intend to weigh yourself at home, buy the most accurate scales you can afford. Average, cheap scales are very approximate as far as small changes in weight are concerned and you cannot rely upon most of them to be consistent.

To get the best out of a pair of bathroom scales, place them on a very firm, uncarpeted surface and mark 'footprints' on them. Adhesive plaster is a convenient way of doing this. Always stand over the 'prints'. Never weigh more frequently than once a day, but once a week is better. Always weigh yourself with an empty bladder and, if possible, after the bowels have moved too. Weigh yourself naked to minimize problems and variations with different clothes. Plot your weight on a weight chart in the bathroom.

Women should pay far less attention to weekly weight changes than men. Fluid retention occurs, to a lesser or greater extent, in all women during their fertile lives. To be sure that you are weighing *you* and not a whole lot of fluid that your body is retaining, you should limit your weigh-ins to the second day of a period.

How fast is weight lost?

The rate of weight-loss is very variable. It is nearly always more rapid at the beginning of a slimming diet. Often, this encouraging start ultimately becomes a reason for failure. A slimmer may suddenly decide after, say, a two-week or month plateau on the weight chart, that the diet is not working. It is important to realize that the very early, rapid weight-loss in most diets is not a fat-loss, but a water-loss. The body gradually readjusts itself and, if you persevere in your chosen diet, fat will be lost relentlessly, if rather slowly.

Keep in mind that your body can never lose weight like a bath losing water when the plug has been taken out. You are too healthy for that to happen. Your body will try its best to retain its 'hard won' fat—after all, it took a long time to gain it. Nevertheless, you will always lose weight if your body is out of energy balance in one way or another (see Chapter XII). Earlier chapters give several examples of how to get yourself into an energy imbalance. When you have chosen your system, stick to it. It will serve you well in the end.

A sensible aim

Chapter I described the latest methods of knowing how fat you are. You will remember that you have to work out a small sum on your pocket calculator. Your weight is divided by your height squared.

A figure of about 20 is normal. Around 25 to 30 you are into mild obesity Grade I. Figures of 30 to 40, Grade II, are worrying, and over 40, Grade III, is positively dangerous. The figure that you calculate for your own height and weight will show you what is a reasonable weight-loss for you and how long you can expect it to take. You may well be able to beat this target by using this book intelligently and going all out on weight reduction. However, you should not be discouraged if you cannot beat this average, slow, but nevertheless relentless weight-loss by dieting.

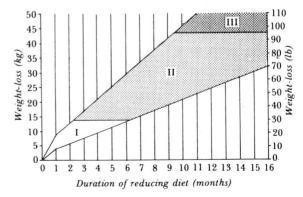

Guide to the length of time it will take on a low-calorie diet to reach the ideal weight.

Tape Measure v. Scales

If you add exercise to your diet regime to achieve that negative energy balance, you will lose *fat* rather quicker than on a diet alone. However, you may also lose *weight* rather slower. There are two reasons for this. All exercise tends to build up muscles and, of course, bigger muscles weigh more than small ones. In addition, exercise often includes a degree of fluid retention (not immediately, but during the days following). You should, therefore, not be obsessive about weighing yourself. Waist, bust and hip measurements will often show fat-loss as fitness better than scales can.

Diets and feeling horrid

Feeling bad while dieting is hardly likely to convince anyone that it is doing him good. Earlier chapters have described how a degree of ketosis complicates many dieting regimes. Fortunately, ketosis is more likely to be experienced as an odd, rather than a nasty, sensation. Most people will tolerate this feeling, if they understand what it is all about and are convinced that it is not at all dangerous. Of course, ketosis is *not* dangerous in any way.

Another complication of some diets is a worn out or 'faint' feeling resulting from 'troughs' of low blood sugar. The wooziness and desolation of low blood sugar, which occurs in the early days of some diets, is less easy to live with. The result is, if somebody feels terrible on a diet, he is most unlikely to persist with it. As explained in Chapter IV, a supply of diet-savers—small packages of carbohydrate foods, like biscuits—is the answer in such cases.

If you look at dieting as a series of self-imposed deprivations, it is unlikely that you will ever win the fight to be slimmer. You will lose a little weight, remain at the new reduced weight for a few weeks and then the scales will start to creep up again. You may even finish up fatter than before. Exercise often helps to promote body awareness, which the diet alone cannot do, and this can help your psychological attitude.

To be permanently successful, all diets must end on a note of permanent change. This may be a change in eating, a change in drinking, a change in exercise patterns or a change in all of them. In effect, a successful dieter has become a changed person, with new eating habits forming part of that change.

Diet-savers

Here are some diet-saving tips to help you survive the occasional moments of weakness.

Often, feeling bad about slimming and dieting is the result of being denied the actual process of chewing, which, for many people, is closely related to the joy of eating. The following diet-savers are very low in calories. In fact, the energy involved in chewing them makes some of them virtually zero calorie gain foods. It is even possible that they actually put you into a negative energy balance, which simply means that you use more energy at a given time than you take in.

Choose from the following list of 100 g (3½ oz) portions:

Cucumber (with salt and pepper)	13 calories
Egg white	16 calories
Lettuce	15 calories
Rhubarb	16 calories
Sauerkraut	16 calories
Tomatoes	19 calories
Tomato juice	19 calories
Watercress	18 calories

Tiny portion foods, even if basically very calorific, are also useful for those who cannot resist the pangs of hunger. Small pickled onions and other vinegar pickles and 1 cm (½ in) cubes of cheese or meat are useful snacks and help to prevent sudden larder raids or to combat an irresistible desire to raid the refrigerator.

Milkless and sugarless tea and coffee have virtually no calorie content.

Zero-calorie fruit drinks sweetened with artificial sweetener will often convince someone that they have had enough to keep them going.

Low calorie sweets can take the edge off the appetite.

A glass of water, a cup of soup or some bran can help to make the stomach feel 'full'.

Eat as many different foods as you can from your diet to avoid feelings of deprivation.

Increase the number of meals that you eat each day, but do not increase the amount of food.

Eat more slowly and take more chews per mouthful.

Eat off a small plate.

A change of occupation often helps. Go out for a walk, do some gardening, write a letter or make a telephone call if you feel hungry.

Quite often small things can distract people from their sensations of hunger, such as putting on a different pair of shoes, changing their clothes, washing their hair.

CHAPTER XII

Diets and exercise

Exercise, together with the diet of your choice, is by far the best way to lose weight. A good walk with the dog, or to the shops, can play a major part in using up calories and keeping you slim.

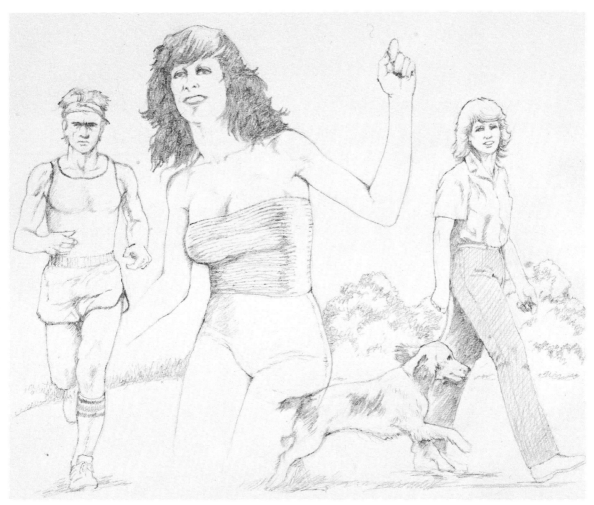

It has been noted in previous chapters how quickly facts are swamped with fallacy as soon as diets and slimming are mentioned. When the loaded word exercise is added, the results are often a web of pure fantasy. Particularly amazing is the use of the same argument to support diametrically opposite views. 'Exercise?' says one, usually failed, dieter, 'rubbish—it just works up an appetite as far as I am concerned', and everyone smiles approvingly. Strangely, the same heads nod their approval when someone says critically 'Of course she's fat, she never moves out of the house'. The true facts provide no support for this anti-exercise propaganda. Admittedly, lumberjacks using up about 6,000 calories a day need to eat more than a clerk clocking up a mere 2,000 or so in the office. However, the clerk will not eat more if he 'works off' an extra 250-350 calories with daily exercise.

Some people, with a scientific turn of mind, are only convinced by unusual experiments, finding those which involve white mice particularly reassuring. Scientists have measured the amount of food eaten by mice that spend quite a lot of time running on tiny treadmills. Compared to mice taking it easy around the cage all day, they tend to eat rather less.

There is, also, an age-old fallacy that fat means lazy. This had been reinforced by the observations of some American workers. They logged the activities of various groups of obese girls, who proved to be far less active than non-obese girls of the same age. However, before a terrible epidemic of 'I told you so' breaks out, consider the work carried out by another group. A pediatrician studied a group of very thin children and compared them to similar fat ones of the same age. It was not the inactivity of the fatter children that impressed him, but the fidgety nature of the thin children. In other words, unless you can make a virtue out of fidgetiness, it is really quite unfair to criticize the obese on the grounds of a quieter disposition and a tendency towards weight gain.

What it cannot do

It is worth knowing what exercise cannot achieve, to avoid wasting time and effort trying the impossible. When very obese people undertake active regimes, such as spending an hour a day on a bicycle pedalometer machine, while maintaining an unrestricted diet, they will lose virtually no weight, even after several weeks. This, of course, does not mean that they are no fitter. They may, in fact, be much fitter in several different ways, but as a method of weight reduction, it will inevitably be a failure.

This simply means that the very obese cannot, apparently, lose weight by exercise alone. Nobody quite knows why this is so. Scientists have, therefore, developed the convenient phrase that obese people are very *resistant* to weight-loss by exercising. It works very well for everyone else, however, as will be shown later in this chapter.

What it can do

Mankind cannot escape the basic laws of thermodynamics. The first law of thermodynamics states quite simply:
Energy balance = Energy intake − Energy expenditure
As fat is the chief energy store in the body, every overweight person has, at some time, been in a positive energy balance. This, sadly, is the very obvious application of Nature's fundamental laws. It must not, however, be twisted or manipulated unfairly when looking at what exercise can do for the slimmer. When food is eaten and utilized by the body, there is always a loss of heat and, therefore, a tendency to move into a negative energy balance. This exists in us all the time. Exercise (by utilization of food) *wastes* energy as well as *producing* energy and so it is basically slimming in itself. The trick is to know how to manipulate exercise in a wasteful way—that is, if it is to be used as a slimming aid.

The anti-exercise stronghold

To a large extent, the conviction that exercise was no use as a slimming aid was a result of doctors being ultra-scientific, or so they thought. They devised experiments in which people did all sorts of energetic things. At the same time, the amount of oxygen they used (burnt) was measured, in an attempt to assess how far they were putting themselves into a negative energy balance. This led to some fairly gloomy forecasts. For instance, it was suggested that to 'exercise off' 450 g (1 lb), you had to play 100 holes on the golf course or 20 sets of tennis or walk about 80 km (50 miles). Understandably, many slimmers lost heart on hearing this and settled for a couple of hours watching sport on the television with a plate of sandwiches and a couple of bottles of beer for consolation.

The good news

The reasons why doctors got it wrong and gave such a bad name to exercise as a slimming aid are now quite well understood. First, measuring gas exchange (oxygen usage or carbon dioxide production) is an unreliable method of looking at energy expenditure in the body. It completely ignores energy expenditure *after* the exercise has stopped (while tissues are being replaced or serviced—a biological process which is in itself very wasteful in energy terms).

The exercise energy forecasters also forgot another important factor. Energy wastage through exercise is cumulative. One scientist, who wanted to find out more about this, pointed out that, if Mr Average spent half an hour a day doing something as relatively low in energy consumption as splitting up firewood, in a year, he would use up the equivalent of 12 kg (26 lb) of body fat.

Another exercise fallacy crept into the popular literature of nutrition some 40 years ago and has still not been fully discredited. Once again, it came from that seemingly impregnable tower of science —white mouse medicine. Mice and rats can be scientifically exercised on treadmills and their weight-loss very accurately measured. In fact, they are very efficient little creatures, as far as energy expenditure is concerned, and they lose very little weight while exercising. One important point was overlooked in this experiment. The energy lost in exercise is related directly to body size and weight. If a rat is exercised for about 10 km (6 miles) per day, the animal uses only about three per cent of his total energy output. When a man walks a similar distance, then ten per cent of his daily (extra) calorie expenditure is produced. An elephant would use up over one-fifth of his daily calorie ration walking a similar distance. In other words, a 10 km (6 mile) walk has quite a part to play in keeping most people slim and using up calories. If taking long walks gets to be a habit with elephants, they could finish up decidedly skinny.

Waste energy to get thin

All the diets in this book have certain advantages to certain people. Choosing the one that suits you best is half the battle, as far as weight reduction is concerned. Choosing the exercise that suits you is also very important. Consider cycling, for example. Many would-be slimmers indulge in spending money as a good substitute for indulging in food. What better way to spend is there than on a nice shiny and expensive bicycle, which seems to invite plenty of exciting, slimming exercise? However, bicycles are really too energy efficient to be very helpful as slimming aids. People with quite severe heart and chest disease, for whom energy expenditure is a burden, find they can cycle more easily than they can walk. The energy expenditure of cycling is about half that used in walking, and a third of that spent in running. Of course, some people are too old or generally too infirm to run, but almost everyone can walk. While half an hour every day spent walking will get you started on a nice little energy expenditure, you will need spend an hour in the saddle to 'waste' as much on your bicycle. You will, of course, travel further, but you could quickly run out of time.

Walk yourself slim

Actually, to get the best out of your 'half hour' walk, you should make it ten minutes longer or, better still, 30 minutes longer. An average 30 minute walk just about uses up the *stored* carbohydrates in the liver and muscles. This is all to the good because they will eventually be made up from the body energy stores (fat). Continuing the walk after the first 30 minutes means that the body switches on to using fat directly as energy and slimming starts in earnest.

Regularity is important in exercise orientated slimming schemes. Two-day programmes are really rather disappointing and your body does need at least a three-day energy boost, however short, before the weighing scales reflect that the laws of thermodynamics are really working in your favour.

Exercise and health

Exercise has very much more to recommend it than simple weight reduction. In every way devised to estimate the health of the heart and lungs, exercise shines through as a health-giving factor. There are several ways of losing weight, but exercise, together with the diet of your choice, is by far the best, as far as health is concerned. It loses fat but not muscle tissue. Lost muscle tissue causes the joints and ligaments to take extra stresses and strains, which are always bad for rheumatism sufferers. Exercise does not cause weight-loss by producing water-loss and subsequent dehydration, unless you go in for playing squash in high temperatures. This form of exercise, although fat-consuming, is suitable only for the very fit and young.

The best exercise

Personal preferences play a major role in the choice of exercise. Jogging has been in vogue in recent years, but it is not necessarily ideal for everyone. The faces of some jogging enthusiasts have a look that suggests stress. There is, undoubtedly, enough stress in the modern world without deliberately inflicting more. However, some people do enjoy jogging and benefit from a regular outing every day. Choose a form of exercise which you find pleasant and which you will, therefore, be likely to 'keep up'.

The best forms of exercise, from the slimming point of view, are those of fairly long duration and those that employ the large muscle groups, such as the legs and shoulder girdles. Anything that involves walking, running, rowing, swimming or dancing is worthwhile. Remember that your body weight will often dictate your exercise schedules and what you can reasonably do, but, for once, you have a built-in bonus. If you are topping the scales at 113 kg (250 lb), as you walk round the golf course, you will spend energy at nearly double the rate of your 68 kg (150 lb) partner (see Chapter VII, exercise chart).

Age-groups and exercise

You should always take whatever exercise you enjoy rather than follow a prescribed routine. Office-bound age-groups may explore isometric exercise systems, which are better than nothing but are not very effective. They are definitely not to be recommended for people with heart or blood

Exercise calories

ACTIVITY	54 kg (120 lb) WOMAN	73 kg (160 lb) MAN
Badminton	90-110	110-130
Basketball	150-200	200-300
Bowling	40-60	50-70
Canoeing	50-75	65-90
Carpentry	50-70	70-90
Cycling (slowly)	50-60	60-70
Cycling (fast)	100-120	140-160
Dancing (ballroom)	50-65	65-85
Dancing (disco)	100-200	125-250
Exercising (not breathless)	70-85	90-110
Exercising (breathless)	100-125	125-175
Football	125-150	150-200
Gardening	60-70	70-90
Golf (1 round)	600-700	700-800
Hockey	125-175	150-200
Jogging	100-125	125-150
Lacrosse	125-175	175-200
Painting and decorating	65-75	75-90
Riding	70-80	80-100
Rowing	150-200	200-250
Running	150-200	200-250
Sawing	125-150	150-200
Skating	100-150	125-175
Skiing (alpine)	100-150	125-175
Squash	90-120	125-200
Swimming	100-150	150-200
Table tennis	75-90	100-125
Tennis	90-110	125-140
Volleyball	90-110	110-140
Walking (stroll)	40-50	45-60
Walking (briskly)	70-80	80-90

pressure problems. The older you get the longer you should exercise because, obviously, the best exercise will not be of a vigorous nature.

The elderly find walking and gardening especially valuable. Not only is there a slimming quotient, but both these activities prevent demineralization of the bone. This is a condition which is quite common in elderly women and can lead to spontaneous bone fractures and broken bones after trivial injuries. The lack of hardness in the bone also compresses it and makes it 'grow downwards'.

Exercise calories

Exercise calorie counting is very variable. Once again, it relies upon Mr and Mrs Average taking part in exercise with an average amount of enthusiasm. This chart shows approximately how many calories are used during 15 minutes of each activity. Clearly, hard playing can increase calorie expenditure considerably, whereas the hang-about on the tennis court who never runs for a ball will probably use fewer calories than shown in the chart. Because of the many individual differences, the figures cannot be precise, but provide general guidelines. It is a good idea to spend at least an extra 300 calories a day as an aid to slimming.

Exercise calorie figures covering a wider range of weights are included in Chapter VII.

The exercise 'hangover'

Never forget those cumulative weight-losses that exercise brings. An extra walk of 1.5 km (1 mile) every day will slim down Mr or Mrs Average by 4.5 kg (10 lb) of fat a year, even if they never open a diet book. Hangovers are usually bad news to everyone, slimmers included, but exercise 'hangovers' are a special benefit.

The exercise 'hangover' is related to the Basic Metabolic Rate. This is the amount of energy needed just to keep the body ticking over—to keep us alive. Doctors measure the B.M.R. in various ways. Usually, to obtain a degree of standardization, they impose strict restrictions on the patient, such as an overnight fast, being at rest and so on. The value obtained—your own B.M.R.—is your tick-over rate of energy expenditure. It represents about a half of your average calorie output in the way of everyday living.

Hardly surprisingly, the B.M.R. changes very rapidly during exercise. However, perhaps the best kept secret of nutrition is that there is a B.M.R. 'hangover' after exercise too. The more vigorous the exercise, the bigger the 'hangover'. A game of football can increase it by 25 per cent, even 15 hours after leaving the playing field, and it is still up 21 per cent six days later!

Fight the flab

'Fight the flab' campaigns are based on the exercise of special muscle groups. It is possible to make thighs and stomachs look better if the flabby fat which they previously carried is converted to (non flabby) muscle. The best abdominal toning exercise is to lie flat on your back on the floor and practise getting yourself into a sitting position. Legs respond well to walking and especially to cycling.

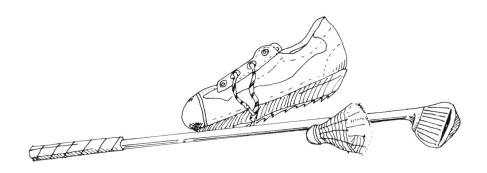

CHAPTER XIII

Special cures

Visiting a health farm or clinic can be a useful, if expensive, aid to weight-loss. Hypnosis is known to work in many cases, but most 'special cures' on offer are only of benefit to the inventor. They separate the slimmer from the pounds in the pocket, not those on the waistline.

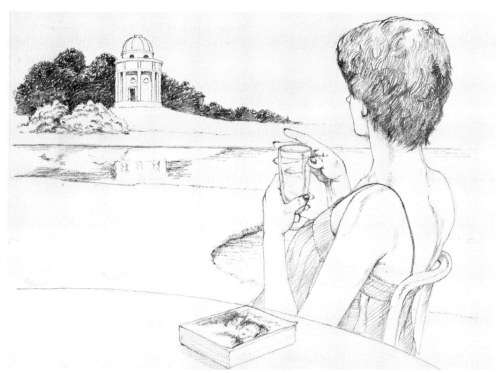

Health farms and clinics have been a growth industry in the last couple of decades. There is no doubt that for people with time and money to spare they can prove a useful aid to weight reduction. Usually they combine a behaviourist approach (see Chapter VII) with a low calorie, largely vegetarian diet. In most clinics alcohol is strictly forbidden and an exercise regime is tailor-made to suit each patient, 'client' or visitor.

Health farms are successful because they involve themselves in the kinds of behaviour alterations that are likely to be followed by weight-loss. Often the environment is luxurious, peaceful and reassuring. Perhaps a large part of the success of health farms is due to the fact that the client is removed from stress and temptation to be self-indulgent, is encouraged to feel better and look better as a direct result of a changed environment, healthy treatments and relaxation, and is allowed to make new and good resolutions relative to a future lifestyle.

Health clinics do vary in the type of fare they provide for their clientele. Would-be slimmers should inquire what sort of dietetic principles they are going to submit to before they part with their fees.

Archetypal in this sort of 'cure' business was a man called Gaylord Hauser. Personally charming, healthy looking and virile, Hauser exploited the 'you too can have a body (and health) like mine' routine to the full and was immensely successful in business. Eventually he could boast a clientele that included Greta Garbo, the Duchess of Windsor, Queen Alexandra of Yugoslavia, Douglas Fairbanks and Norma Shearer.

His technique was simple. He ran health clinics and he also invented and manufactured an impressive range of health foods. Once a week his non-clinic patients had to retire from everyday life and exist on Hauser patent foods only. These included such therapeutic boons as Hollywood Slimming Tea, Healthwise Sipp and Nu-veg-Sal. It seems that most of these were low-calorie products and all that happened was that Hauser's clients followed a near starvation routine one day in seven. For those who habitually over-ate, the results could well have been beneficial.

Gaylord Hauser's successful slimming cures relied on a personality cult and a modicum of trickery. However, more seriously, slimming cures of a devious and dangerous nature persist.

Hormones and diets

For years there have been enthusiasts for hormone-aided diets. Many years ago, thyroid hormones were used and, more recently, injections of sex hormones. The consensus of informed medical opinion is that such treatments are dangerous and/or totally useless. They should definitely be avoided.

The fat actress

An echo from the past which has not quite died away is the story of Texas Guinan and Walter C. Cunningham. Before starting in the mail order slimming business, Cunningham had graduated through the hard school of fraudulent property business. He was, perhaps, the first person to realize the power of personality when it comes to selling a dietetic 'miracle'. As an ex-convict and crook, his own personality was not particularly attractive, so he hit on the idea of buying one that was. He formed a partnership with Texas Guinan, an actress whose talents had been overlooked by Broadway and Hollywood.

Early advertisements for the Texas Guinan world-famed treatment for obesity told a sad tale of the ruin of her promising career in the theatre. One day, her agent had put his arm around her sadly, led her to the door of his office and affectionately shown her out. The reasons for this lack of enthusiasm for Miss Guinan had nothing to do with her acting ability, the story goes. There was no evidence of temperamental behaviour, or even alcoholism. Her problem was obesity. As Texas herself said, 'In tights I was a sight at 204 pounds.' We can agree with this judgment, for she published a photograph that proved it.

Texas's story was that in her desolation she came across Walter Cunningham's obesity cure— and tried it. Within 10 days, she lost 8 kg (17½ lb). 'Joy returned,' she told the readers of Cunningham's advertisements. 'I was found dancing before the mirror, singing as a full throated lark sings at dawn.' Naturally, she returned to her theatrical agent who made her an 'offer that made her eyes stick out'. Exactly what this offer was is not specified, but, by now, Miss Guinan felt, she tells us, that she had another calling of greater meaning than the tinsel attractions of a life on the boards. Instead, she decided to devote her considerable talents to the easement of the profound psychological and physical suffering of the obese.

The American Medical Association, however, was not totally convinced of Texas's self-sacrifice and idealism. They knew of her association with the gaol-bird Cunningham and looked unkindly upon his patent medicine company which manufactured the nostrum that rescued Miss Guinan

from her plight. What is more, they started replying to the Guinan positive fat reducer advertisements for further information and advice.

The results were predictable. In response to the first enquiry, the cure was offered at a mere twenty dollars, a considerable sum in those days. The AMA did not send the money and soon received a second letter from Texas offering the obesity cure at half price. Still the AMA hardened their hearts and a third letter arrived from Miss Guinan. She was disappointed, naturally, but still offered the chance for the AMA to attain a 'pliant reed-like form—the glory of youth's lithesome grace'. A fourth letter offered the cure for a 'mere five dollars' and letter number five further reduced the fee to three dollars.

At this point, the AMA decided to subscribe to the therapeutic boon that would 'render your chin, throat, arms, abdomen, hips, thighs and lower limbs—enchanting'. The mixture was a muddy liquid consisting of alum, alcohol and water, devoid of therapeutic effects in the slimming or any other field. Later, a Los Angeles judge issued a fraud order against Texas Guinan Incorporated and a profitable 'obesity cure' disappeared, only to be remembered as an example of ingenious mail order quackery.

Reducing salts and saunas

Although the hey-day of bogus obesity cures was in the 1920s and 1930s, quite a lot of the convincing patter remains in the slimming business. In the past, special reducing salts, some of which you ate, some of which you put in the bath, held great sway. Today, the slimming effects of such nostrums are rarely advertised, other than by word of mouth. They are all, of course, quite useless. Certain 'health salts', such as Epsom salts and Glauber's salt, will cause a temporary weight reduction due to dehydration —water loss from the body. The modern equivalent for temporary dehydration is, of course, the sauna. Disappointingly and quite predictably, the weight goes back on again as soon as the slimmer has drunk enough liquid to rehydrate his or her body.

Creams and massage

Another big seller in the slimming field included various pastes and ointments, advertised as dissolving away fat or as creating that therapeutic nirvana so much desired by beauty writers the world over, so-called 'spot slimming'. Regrettably, it has long been established that this weight-loss, as a result of the use of such nostrums, will only come about as a result of a lightening of the purse and pocket.

Mechanical aids

Closely related to, and sometimes combined with, 'rub off fat' cures are various mechanical devices marketed as slimming aids. Again, sensible advertising control has reduced the impact of such paraphernalia and prevents false claims being made. However, the wily merchant can often find a way of promoting such inventions, while remaining within the letter of the law. For example, various devices for the treatment of an obesity-related condition, called *cellulite*, are currently very fashionable. It is difficult to decide whether any of the *cellulite* therapies really 'works', because no one can define accurately exactly what *cellulite* is.

Beauty experts think they know about *cellulite* and talk of strange accumulations of fat or fluid in the subcutaneous tissues, mostly in the legs, of women. Reputable dermatologists deny its existence and unkindly describe it instead as 'localized fat deposits', which give the *cellulite* appearance to the flabby legs and thighs of sufferers. Fat is deposited in various, fairly well-defined areas in the skin, although these differ somewhat between the sexes. Significantly, very slim people never seem to suffer from *cellulite*. The only thing that any machine, belt, special corset or vibration device can do, as far as fat is concerned, is to push it around temporarily. They have nothing at all to do with effective slimming.

Electric current stimulation

Electric current stimulation is another pretty ineffective slimming aid. Muscles are made to contract by using electricity, but it is perfectly easy to contract those very muscles by Nature. Converting flabby fat to muscle is the essence of the 'fight the flab' campaigns, based on exercising special muscle groups.

Hypnosis

Hypnosis has been defined as 'a temporary condition of altered attention, the most striking feature of which is increased suggestibility. Hypnosis has something in common with sleep but, once hypnotized, the subject is in a condition very unlike sleep. The mind is concentrated and the body works, in terms of physical responses, rather as it does while awake. In a nutshell, hypnosis is a third state of mind between wakefulness and sleep.

The extent to which hypnosis can help people change their behaviour (in our case, alter their eating patterns) is very variable and to understand this properly it is necessary to mention hysteria. When doctors talk about hysteria they refer to something very different to the sort of thing we label as 'hysterical' in everyday parlance, when 'hystrionic' would be the better word to use. In medical terminology, a patient's anxiety about a basic conflict (e.g. he is far too fat but cannot get thin) may be converted into a symptom which usually carries what is called 'a secondary gain'. This secondary gain somehow solves the patient's dilemma in hysteria.

An extreme example of secondary gain is that of a man who found out that while he was at work his wife was visiting her lover. He developed hysterical paralysis of the legs. He could not go to work and his wife lost her clandestine opportunities. Secondary gain situations in slimming are quite common and umpteen reasons (symptoms) are produced by people to prevent them adhering to a sensible slimming routine. These symptoms include weakness, tiredness, fainting, lack of concentration, palpitations and nerves.

Hysterical personalities are very prone to suggestion and therefore to hypnosis therapy. People can be helped, by means of hypnosis, to start slimming and also to stop smoking. It is important to differentiate between lay and medical hypnosis. Although there are good, even excellent, lay hypnotists, there is now an Association of Medical Hypnotists and I, personally, believe that a good, medically qualified hypnotist is better than a lay hypnotist when it comes to helping someone who wishes to use hypnosis as a slimming aid.

It is possibly unwise to dismiss the concept of hysteria, referred to briefly above, quite so simplistically. Hysteria may take many forms. Hysterical loss of memory is well-known. It may be manifest as a disorder of consciousness. Disorders of mobility are far from rare and some obese people are made to feel so 'ill' by exercise that their chances of success in slimming are small. Hysterical disorders of perception (e.g. blindness and deafness) are rare but other strange disorders of 'feeling' are quite common.

CHAPTER XIV

Staying slim and healthy

Once the extra weight is shed, the diet which worked for you should continue to be followed in a modified form. High fibre diets and certain special diets can also contribute to keeping the family slim and healthy.

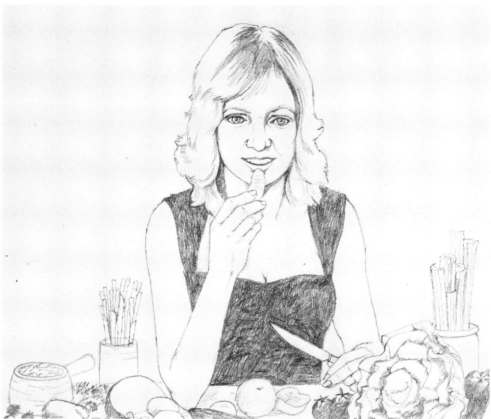

Having reached an ideal weight, maintaining it is the name of the game and all successful diets need a constant injection of top-up enthusiasm. The late Dr Tarnower, who had such success with his Scarsdale Medical Diet (see Chapter VIII), sensibly placed great reliance on his Keep Trim Programme. *How to be a lifetime winner* was another of these themes.

How to be a lifetime winner

The Scarsdale Keep Trim Programme is a simple modification of the basic Scarsdale low fat, low carbohydrate, high protein diet, but not so confining. Once the target weight is reached the Keep Trim diet can be modified by, say, an alcoholic drink a day, extra meat or fish, a few more eggs, more cheese, a few slices of bread. Weight changes must be carefully noted over the next two weeks. If weight increases then less extra foods are allowed the following week. If weight loss continues or is maintained, extra food may be taken.

Part of the Tarnower credo is to admit that most overweight people love their food. This is

how they became obese. Dr Tarnower suggested to his patients that they should take a leaf or two out of the book of the wine connoisseur who examines, admires, criticizes the colour and bouquet of the wine, sniffs the cork, savours the taste and then sips lovingly and slowly, enjoying every drop. Food, it is suggested, should be treated in the same way. It should be prepared with loving respect and eaten slowly, with plenty of chewing. Scarsdale acolytes are encouraged to develop a state of mind that means that they can prepare and eat a plate of scrambled eggs with as much enthusiasm and delight as a steak and kidney pudding. This post-diet regime lays a lot of stress on garnishes and attractive food presentation. Once prepared, the food is enjoyed over as long a period as possible. Doubtless for those who can accept the Scarsdale philosophy of eating, it works very well.

Diet maintenance

In more practical, everyday home slimming terms, diet maintenance is perhaps less heady in its concept than Dr Tarnower's Scarsdale philosophy, but it must be based on a continuance in a modified form of the dietary system that has worked for you. This eating pattern should be followed on a lifetime basis. Men should weigh themselves once every two weeks. Women, during their fertile years, should check their weight on the same day of their menstrual cycle each month. After the menopause they, too, can weigh-in every two weeks. An increase in weight indicates that a diet adjustment is necessary and the original diet should be closely followed until the target weight is regained.

High fibre diet

Increasing gradually the fibre content of the food you eat, with an emphasis on natural, unprocessed foods, can make a great contribution to a 'keep slim and healthy' campaign in the family.

Fibre recipes are far from dull, as those which follow will show. Fibre is a valuable slimming aid and helps in several ways. High fibre foods have fewer calories and greater bulk than the same amount of low fibre or highly refined food. They need more chewing and this gives them a high satiety value. In addition, the actual 'work' done in chewing also helps to establish a regulative energy balance.

There is some evidence that high fibre foods act rather like a sponge, retaining fluid and reducing the amount of energy absorbed from food. Less energy absorbed means that foods are less fattening and some dietary experts argue that high fibre diets reduce the (useful) calorific value of foods quite profoundly.

Fibre foods contain different amounts of fibre and varying numbers of calories. The WHAT IS IN FOOD tables in Chapter III show the weights of dietary fibre and the calories per 100 g (3½ oz) of food. Breakfast cereals, such as All-Bran and Puffed Wheat, crispbread and wholemeal bread are good sources of fibre.

High fibre recipes

Fruit and Nut Slaw
SERVES 6

150 ml (5 fl oz) low fat yogurt
225 g (8 oz) white cabbage, finely shredded
2 large carrots, grated
1 green apple, thinly sliced
juice of ½ lemon
75 g (3 oz) sultanas
25 g (1 oz) walnuts, chopped
½ teaspoon paprika

Mix all the ingredients together until they are thoroughly combined. Chill in the refrigerator for 1 hour before serving.

Fried Heart with Parsley
SERVES 4

450 g (1 lb) heart (beef, pig or lamb)
2 tablespoons wholemeal flour
2 tablespoons corn oil
2 garlic cloves, crushed
juice of 2 lemons
75 g (3 oz) wholemeal breadcrumbs
4 tablespoons chopped, fresh parsley

Cut the heart into thin strips about 6mm (¼ in) thick. Coat the strips with the flour, shaking off any excess.

Heat the oil in a frying-pan. Add the heart strips and the garlic. Cook, stirring frequently, for 6-8 minutes.

Remove the heart and garlic from the pan. Set aside and keep warm.

Add the lemon juice to the pan. Stir in the breadcrumbs and 3 tablespoons of parsley. Return the heart slices to the pan and cook, stirring and tossing, until they are well coated with the breadcrumb and parsley mixture.

Transfer to a serving dish, sprinkle over the remaining parsley and serve immediately.

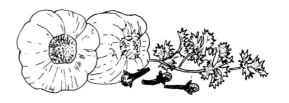

Potato and Carrot Cake
SERVES 6

1 tablespoon plus 1 teaspoon corn oil
1 small onion, peeled and chopped
225 g (8 oz) carrots, sliced
225 g (8 oz) potatoes, scrubbed and sliced
2 teaspoons chopped, fresh sage
75 g (3 oz) wholemeal flour
1 teaspoon baking powder
salt and pepper
1 tablespoon chopped, fresh chives

Preheat the oven to 220°C (425°F), gas mark 7. Lightly grease a baking sheet with 1 teaspoon of corn oil and set aside.

Heat the remaining oil in a frying-pan. Add the onion and cook, stirring occasionally, for 5-7 minutes, or until it is soft and translucent. Remove the pan from the heat and set aside.

Put the carrots and potatoes in a large saucepan and pour over sufficient boiling water to cover. Simmer for 10-15 minutes, or until the vegetables are tender.

Drain the carrots and potatoes and transfer them to a mixing bowl. Mash thoroughly. Add the onion, sage, flour, baking powder and salt and pepper to taste. Mix well until all the ingredients are thoroughly combined and form a dough.

Turn the dough out on to a lightly floured board. Roll it into a circle, about 20 cm (8 in) in diameter. Mark with a knife into 6 wedges and transfer to the prepared baking sheet.

Bake for 30 minutes, or until the cake has risen and is golden brown. Sprinkle over the chives and serve immediately.

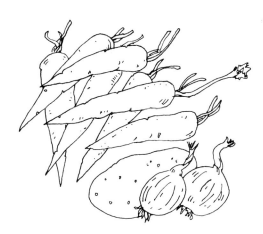

Polish Cabbage
SERVES 6

900 g (2 lb) red cabbage, shredded
1 tablespoon corn oil
1 large onion, peeled and sliced
50 g (2 oz) wholemeal flour
75 ml (3 fl oz) wine vinegar
1 tablespoon brown sugar

Put the cabbage in a large saucepan and pour over sufficient boiling water to cover. Boil for 10 minutes.

Drain the cabbage and reserve 850 ml (1½ pints) of the cooking liquid. Set the cabbage and reserved liquid aside.

Heat the oil in a frying-pan. Add the onion and fry, stirring occasionally, for 5-7 minutes, or until it is soft and translucent. Add the flour and cook, stirring constantly, for 1 minute.

Remove the pan from the heat. Gradually stir in 575 ml (1 pint) of the reserved cooking liquid to make a smooth sauce.

Mix together the cabbage, the sauce, the vinegar and sugar. Transfer to a large saucepan and set the pan over low heat. Cook, stirring occasionally, for 1½ hours. If necessary, add a little of the remaining reserved cooking liquid from time to time to prevent sticking.

Brown Rice Salad
SERVES 6

3 tablespoons wine vinegar
3 tablespoons sunflower seed oil
juice of 1 orange
225 g (8 oz) long grain brown rice, cooked, drained and kept warm
2 oranges, peeled and divided into segments
1 tablespoon chopped, fresh chives
1 celery stalk, chopped
50 g (2 oz) sultanas
75 g (3 oz) peanuts
75 g (3 oz) aduki beans, soaked overnight and drained

Beat together the vinegar, oil and orange juice. Pour 75 ml (3 fl oz) of the mixture over the warm rice and stir to mix well. Set aside to cool to room temperature.

Stir in the oranges, chives, celery, sultanas, peanuts, beans and the remaining dressing. Cover and chill in the refrigerator for 1 hour before serving.

Seafood Hotpot
SERVES 4-6

1 tablespoon corn oil
2 large onions, peeled and thinly sliced
2 garlic cloves, crushed
25 g (1 oz) wholemeal flour
275 ml (10 fl oz) dry, white wine
juice of ½ lemon
700 g (1½ lb) white fish fillets, cut into chunks
450 g (1 lb) potatoes, unpeeled and thinly sliced
125 g (4 oz) prawns
75 g (3 oz) mushrooms, sliced
225 g (8 oz) tomatoes, coarsely chopped
2 tablespoons chopped, fresh parsley
½ lemon, thinly sliced

Preheat the oven to 180°C (350°F), gas mark 4.

Heat the oil in a frying-pan. Add the onions and garlic and cook, stirring occasionally, for 5-7 minutes, or until they are soft and translucent.

Add the flour and cook, stirring constantly, for 1 minute. Remove the pan from the heat. Gradually stir in the wine and the lemon juice. Return the pan to the heat and cook, stirring constantly, for 2 minutes. Remove the pan from the heat and set aside.

Mix together the onion and sauce mixture, the fish and the potatoes.

Reserve 4-6 prawns for garnish. Shell and devein the remainder. Stir the shelled prawns into the fish mixture. Add the mushrooms and tomatoes. Transfer the mixture to an ovenproof casserole, cover and bake for 1 hour.

Garnish the casserole with the reserved prawns, the parsley and the lemon slices and serve immediately.

Country Quiche
SERVES 6

225 g (8 oz) wholemeal flour
125 g (4 oz) butter
125 g (4 oz) Cheddar cheese, grated
2-4 tablespoons cold water
Filling:
12 spring onions
225 g (8 oz) tomatoes, chopped and drained
1 tablespoon chopped, fresh parsley
75 g (3 oz) Cheddar cheese, grated
2 eggs, lightly beaten
150 ml (5 fl oz) milk
salt and pepper
15 g (½ oz) Parmesan cheese, grated

Preheat the oven to 200°C (400°F), gas mark 6.

Put the flour and butter into a mixing bowl. Cut the butter into the flour and then rub it in, using the fingertips, until the mixture resembles coarse breadcrumbs. Stir in the cheese. Make a well in the centre and gradually add sufficient water to make a firm dough.

Turn the dough out on to a lightly floured board. Roll it out into a circle large enough to line a 23 cm (9 in) flan tin. Ease the dough circle into the flan tin and transfer the tin to a baking sheet. Line the pastry case with foil or greaseproof paper and weigh it down with pieces of bread or dried beans.

Bake for 15 minutes. Remove the bread or beans and the foil or greaseproof paper. Continue baking for 5-10 minutes, or until the pastry case is just beginning to turn brown.

Remove the pastry case from the oven and set aside. Reduce the oven temperature to 180°C (350°F), gas mark 4.

Trim 4 spring onions and set aside. Cut the remaining spring onions into slices and mix together with the tomatoes, parsley and Cheddar cheese. Arrange the mixture over the bottom of the pastry case and set aside.

Beat the eggs and milk together and add salt and pepper to taste. Pour the egg and milk mixture into the pastry case.

Arrange the reserved spring onions decoratively on top and sprinkle over the Parmesan cheese.

Bake the quiche for 25-30 minutes, or until it is set and lightly browned.

Serve immediately, if serving hot, or set aside to cool to room temperature, if serving cold.

Fruit Salad
SERVES 6

2 oranges, peeled and coarsely chopped
2 red-skinned dessert apples, thinly sliced
2 bananas, peeled and sliced
1 pear, peeled and chopped
225 g (8 oz) strawberries, hulled and halved
125 g (4 oz) grapes, halved and seeded
1 peach, peeled, stoned and sliced
250 ml (10 fl oz) fresh orange juice

Mix together all the fruit and pour over sufficient orange juice to cover. Chill in the refrigerator for 1 hour before serving.

(Recipes compiled by Drs Penny and Andrew Stanway for the manufacturers of Fybogel)

Diets to keep you healthy

Most doctors would shake their heads if asked whether it were possible to select a diet to keep you healthy, but some would nod enthusiastically. Although there is little scientific theory to support the claim that the following diets are exceptionally effective, some people swear by them.

Diet for a good complexion

Over-consumption of all foods is prohibited and emphasis is given to plenty of protein in the diet. These rules should be followed.
1 **Don't eat any fat (butter, margarine, cream, whole milk or whole milk cheeses). Cottage cheese is allowed and so is skimmed milk.**
2 **Don't eat chocolates or sweets.**
3 **Don't eat fried or highly seasoned foods.**
4 **Don't eat mayonnaise.**
5 **Don't eat pies or pizzas.**
6 **Drink sugar-free drinks only.**
7 **Don't drink alcohol.**

Anti allergy diets

These diets obviously avoid specific foods known to produce allergic reactions. They are based on 'Stone Age' dietary principles and the dieter must imagine himself, or herself, back in the Stone Age living on what Nature can provide in the way of hunted or gathered foods. In other words, the dieter must follow an unrefined carbohydrate diet. Natural carbohydrates and natural foods are allowed but clearly all manufactured, processed and canned foods are taboo. The Stone Age diet makes considerable demands on the food preparer and, to start with, the palate. Many people, however, find that their allergies as well as their obesity will disappear on such a regime.

Anti rheumatoid diet

People who suffer from certain types of rheumatoid arthritis, who are also overweight, will benefit from weight reduction. Rheumatoid arthritis is a disease characterized by remissions and exacerbations. During the latter phase when the joints are swollen, Dr Irwin M. Stillman, a physician from Coney Island, New York, recommends a diet rich in Vitamin B and low in sodium compounds. It is also low in calories.

High B complex foods include wholewheat and wheatgerm products. Low salt foods include beans, cabbage, cranberries, grapefruit, grapes, lemons, plums and melon.

A typical day's menu for a person on an anti rheumatoid diet would be as follows.

BREAKFAST
1 slice wholemeal bread
1 egg
Tea or coffee

LUNCH
125 g (4 oz) meat, chicken, fish or
  1 egg
125 g (4 oz) rice
½ tomato
Tea or coffee

DINNER
Vegetable soup
50 g (2 oz) meat
125 g (4 oz) rice
Tea or coffee

A Vitamin B complex capsule should be taken daily. Wheatgerm can be sprinkled over breakfast cereal.

Gall bladder diet

A low fat diet (see Chapter VIII) keeps gall bladder symptoms at bay in many cases. Sufferers are frequently overweight and if normal weight is reached the symptoms often disappear. The weight reduction achieved by a high protein, low calorie, low fat diet also allows gall bladder surgery to be carried out, should it become necessary, with minimum risk and followed by a quick convalescence.

Gout diet

Gout diets are designed to limit the intake of food in conjunction with medical advice. These rules should be followed.
1 **Avoid totally salmon, tuna, smoked fish, anchovies, sweetbreads, kidney, brains, liver, meat extracts, chocolates, nuts, salad dressing, coffee, cocoa and alcohol.**
2 **Limit allowed meat to 125 g (4 oz) per day.**
3 **Eat 1 egg per day.**
4 **Eat small portions of lentils, beans, spinach or peas daily.**
5 **Eat up to three slices of bread daily.**

CHAPTER XV

Questions and answers

This chapter covers a wide range of subjects of interest to the slimmer and draws on recent medical research taking place in Europe and America.

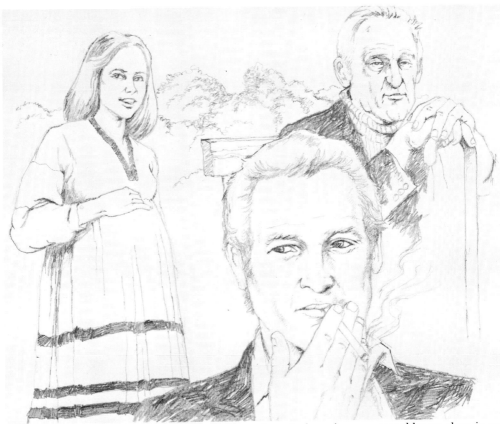

Questions on diets and slimming are often asked and this chapter answers many of them. It also gives an opportunity to discuss in more detail some of the topics mentioned in earlier chapters.

Calories

Question   What is a calorie?

Answer   A calorie is a heat unit. It is the amount of heat required to raise the temperature of 1 g of water through 1° Centigrade. This is the calorie of the physicist. Nutritionists find that if they use these small calories, food values finish up with strings of noughts after them. They use the great Calorie, or Kilocalorie, which equals 1,000 small calories. The calories referred to in books on food and dieting are always Kilocalories.

Joules

Question   What is a joule?

Answer   A joule is a measure of energy. Mr Joule was a physicist who wished to express the amount of work done in one second by an electric current of 1 ampere against a resistance of 1 ohm. A joule is the equivalent of heat (or work converted to heat) that will raise the temperature of 1 g of water by 1° Centigrade. A joule is equal to one small calorie.

Overweight and glands

Question   How much has obesity to do with glands? I've heard lots of theories and I think it is my glands, because I really eat very little, yet remain overweight despite dieting.

Answer   This matter was briefly discussed in Chapter III. In fact, there are relatively few glandular conditions associated with overweight.

Myxoedema, a disease of the thyroid gland, is the commonest example. For some reason, the thyroid fails to function, but this happens so slowly that victims often do not realize what is happening to them.

In the early stages, the sufferer complains of the cold and seems to be slowing up mentally. Often the muscles ache and sometimes numbness and tingling feelings occur too. The memory gradually deteriorates and reactions become much slower. Constipation may well develop. Women's voices become lower in pitch and abnormalities of menstruation are common. The skin becomes rather dry, the hair tends to thin (especially the outer one-third of the eyebrows) and weight-gain occurs relentlessly, in spite of strict dieting.

Diagnosis is often delayed because of the gradual onset of the illness, but is quite easily clinched by means of blood tests and, sometimes, by measuring the metabolic rate. Treatment is dramatic and effective. Thyroid hormone is given on a regular basis—for life. The symptoms disappear and weight returns to normal.

Myxoedema is the only reason for a doctor to prescribe thyroid tablets. In the past, they were sometimes given as a slimming aid. It is now known that, apart from the treatment of myxoedema, this is both dangerous and ineffective.

Another glandular cause of obesity is Cushing's syndrome. This is caused by an oversecretion of two small glands, the adrenal glands, situated over the kidneys. Again, the onset is gradual, but takes several months rather than several years. Early symptoms are generalized weakness and lassitude, weight-gain, backache and a rounding of the face. Some women become excessively hairy and periods cease. Men may become impotent. The skin tends to bruise easily and acne often develops. The obesity is of a rather special type—the trunk becomes fat, but the arms and legs remain slender. Often, stretch marks (striae) appear on the hips, tummy, flanks and around the armpit folds.

Cushing's disease needs urgent investigation and treatment. With satisfactory management both the obesity and the disease itself can be well controlled.

The third glandular cause of obesity is the menopause, or change of life, when yet other glands, the ovaries, stop working. Compared with the previous conditions, the link between the menopause and obesity is not so well marked.

There is a theory that the change of life in itself has no effect on weight-gain. It is claimed that the obesity which often complicates it is always due to overeating as a form of compensation. In other words, women are so upset by 'losing their femininity' at the menopause that they comfort themselves with food.

There is no doubt at all that weight-gain is common at the menopause, but the theory of compensation does not seem very satisfactory.

Only a few women, about five to ten per cent, experience a bad menopause or are unduly upset by it. Some, about ten per cent, hardly notice it at all, except that their periods stop. The rest experience a transient upset in their lifestyles, mainly because the circulatory system becomes unstable. Hot flushes and palpitations are common and life temporarily loses its general tranquillity.

Although statistical evidence is lacking, it seems that more women gain weight at the change of life than are upset by that change. The middle-aged spread of women may in fact have glandular components to it. Tiresome menopausal symptoms are reasonably easily controlled these days. Unfortunately, treatment, even hormone replacement therapy, does not remedy the obesity. To do that, you must follow the general principles of slimming in the earlier chapters of this book.

Constant weight v. fatten easily

Question Is it true that some people burn off fat more easily than others?

Answer It would be very neat if, after dealing with the two, or possibly three, real *glandular* causes of obesity, we could sit back and say that is that. In other words, you just get fat by overeating. In fact, most doctors and dieticians have been saying just that for many years. However, there is quite a lot of evidence that metabolic, if not glandular, factors play an important role in obesity. Metabolism is the shorthand name for all the build-up and breakdown of the body, going on all day and every day and it is closely linked with many of the glands in our bodies. Thus, a new glandular theory about obesity becomes very likely.

To provide a standard measurement, metabolic rate is defined as the rate of energy expenditure under conditions of complete relaxation, after a 12-hour fast. To eliminate all variables, the environmental temperature is pegged at 28°C (82.4°F). At this temperature, the body does not have to expend variable amounts of energy to keep warm. The metabolic rate, therefore, accounts for the energy used by the body's constant building and replacement of tissues, together with various inner mechanical energy expenditure, such as the heart's action. In other words, the metabolic rate is equivalent to the energy we use just to keep us alive. Furthermore, it accounts for

55-60 per cent of our average daily energy expenditure. This is quite a large proportion, especially in comparison to the energy cost of average physical activity, which is only about 20 per cent of daily energy expenditure. Clearly, variations in metabolic rate play quite a large part in maintaining our energy balance when we stay at a constant weight, or imbalance when we increase or decrease in weight.

When thyroid hormone is used to treat myxoedema, the obesity melts away due to the resultant increase in the metabolic rate. It would be splendid, if we had a 'pill' at our disposal, which would do the same thing to the metabolic rate of the obese person not suffering from myxoedema. Unfortunately, we do not. Nevertheless, what little we do know about variations in metabolic rate is news for slimmers and also helps to explain why slimming is a difficult task, especially for certain age groups.

Unfortunately, the metabolic rate tends to decrease with weight-loss. This is probably an example of Nature trying to be helpful. Nature seems to have a vested interest in keeping us plump, perhaps for survival in times of famine, and reacts to weight-loss by lowering the metabolic rate in the Fatten Easilies. The table (below) shows what happened to the metabolic rates of a group of middle-aged women, who are now at normal weight but who were previously obese.

Although ways of altering the Basic Metabolic Rate for slimmers are limited at the moment, research shows that the future outlook could be rosier. Researchers at Cambridge have found that a substance, known as T_3, can help slimmers who get stuck at a no weight-loss period, usually after four to six weeks of dieting. It seems that, during severely restricted dieting, the body's own T_3 production falls and this reduces the metabolic rate. In other words, the body 'tries' to keep its weight static. Not all 'stuck' dieters, however, respond to T_3.

Metabolic rate may seem depressing news to some slimmers, now that they understand how a few hundred extra calories a day are turned into stored fat in the recently slimmed. However, mathematically minded slimmers will perk up when they realize that the energy expenditure sums are not yet complete.

> Basic Metabolic Rate =
>   55-60% of calorie expenditure
> Normal exercise =
>   20% of calorie expenditure
> Remainder =
>   20-25% of calorie expenditure

This unaccounted for 20-25 per cent of calorie expenditure is well worth the slimmer's interest.

It is likely that what metabolic experts call *thermogenic* (heat generated) *components* of energy expenditure account for these 'missing' calories. Several factors operate together to make up the total thermogenic component. It is fashionable to separate these factors and look at the total thermogenic components thus:

> Thermogenic components (total) =
> Non shivering thermogenesis
> Meal induced thermogenesis
> Drug induced thermogenesis
> Psychologically induced thermogenesis

Not a great deal is known about drug induced and psychological thermogenesis. They certainly have an effect, but we do not understand it very well. It is better, therefore, not to pin too many hopes on it, although at least one 'slimming pill' bases part of its action on drug induced thermogenesis.

Two commonly used drugs—caffeine and tobacco—do produce and increase thermogenesis. Coffee plays a major part in many popular slimming diets and people who give up smoking often put on weight for several months.

Non shivering thermogenesis is exactly what it says—heat production induced without the involvement of shivering. Recent research has

Basic Metabolic Rate

B.M.R. of nine women

	Weight when obese	Present weight	Present percentage above ideal	Present age (years)	Present Basic Metabolic Rate	Ideal Basic Metabolic Rate
Mean	83.2 kg (184 lb)	67.4 kg (148 lb)	15.9	47.3	5.38	5.92

shown that NST, as it is called, accounts for one particular type of obesity in experimental animals. It may also have a bearing on the obesity of humans, which takes us back to our old friend, Mrs Fatten Easily.

It is possible to breed a mouse that very quickly becomes obese. After weaning and despite eating a normal amount of food, it becomes obese quite quickly, *but only if its body temperature falls below normal*. Otherwise, this 'genetic' factor does not operate and the mouse does not become obese. This neatly demonstrates the interplay between genetic factors and what happens to weight-gain in differing circumstances. The genetically 'obese mouse', living in an average mouse environment, can virtually halve its energy losses. It does this by reducing its non shivering thermogenesis. Thus, it rapidly becomes a really nice, fat, little mouse, by turning food into stored fat.

There are warnings elsewhere in this book against too ready an application of white, or any other type of, mouse medicine to Man. However, in this case of non shivering thermogenesis, human experiments, mostly part of cold- adaptation studies, show that those with a built-in propensity to obesity have a non shivering thermogenesis profile similar to that of genetically obese mice. At 20°C (68°F) lean people have no trouble in maintaining their inner 'core' temperature. Perhaps surprisingly, the obese show a rapid fall in their deep 'core' temperature. It is likely that these differences are related to metabolic rate. Lean people can switch the rate up quite rapidly, but the obese cannot and so they quickly cool down.

Working alongside non shivering thermogenesis is meal-induced thermogenesis. For nearly 80 years, nutritionists have been trying to explain Mr Constant Weight, who simply does not get fat. After they have overeaten, the calories are dissipated as excess heat. Nutritionists have called this *luxus consumption*.

It is well known that the metabolic rate increases on eating. It is quite easy to understand why there is a peak in the rate after a meal—the digestion, absorption and redistribution of nutrients all cost energy. Certain foods, notably protein, seem to be particularly liable to produce heat in this way, although the reasons for this are not understood.

This raises an important question. Does Mrs Fatten Easily have a lower built-in power of luxus consumption than Mr Constant Weight?

If so, this would help to explain why they gain weight more easily when they overeat, even just occasionally. Although little convincing research has been done on this subject, low-power luxus consumption does seem to be linked with obesity.

The 'organ' responsible for controlling both non shivering thermogenesis and luxus consumption has only recently been identified as the brown adipose tissue, or brown fat. This is now revealing clues to some of the puzzles of obesity. The amount of brown fat in the body increases in response to cold environments. How much, therefore, is obesity related to the temperature of our houses and offices or even to the clothes we wear?

Brown fat appears to be the slimmer's dream and the gourmet's delight. It effectively bypasses the normal chain of events in which excess calories consumed are reflected in excess weight recorded on the scales. Anything we can do to enhance its production will reduce obesity and ideas along these lines may be the slimming methods of the future. At the moment, all that can be said with certainty, as far as 'wasting' calories is concerned is that, in terms of brown fat, four hints tip the balance in favour of slimming.

1 **Small frequent meals.**
2 **High protein diets.**
3 **Lower ambient temperatures and, perhaps, fewer clothes.**
4 **Caffeine and smoking.**

Pregnancy and breastfeeding

Question Should I diet during pregnancy or when I am breastfeeding?

Answer Yes, you should diet if you are overweight. Good pregnancy and feeding nutrition is worked out around a simple list of rules.

1 **Forget about the saying, 'you are eating for two'.**
2 **Each day, drink not less than 575 ml (1 pint) of milk, and eat not less than two eggs and a 125-g (4-oz) portion of fish, offal, cheese, bacon or good quality processed meat.**
3 **Each day, eat no more than 75 g (3 oz) wholemeal bread, two good-sized portions of beans or lentils, carrots, peas, parsnips or turnip.**
4 **Eat as much as you like of fresh fruit, without sugar, greens and salads, celery and bran.**
5 **Try to avoid sugar, too much salt, processed carbohydrates, junk foods and alcohol.**

Overweight when pregnant

Question   How do you know if you are overweight during pregnancy?

Answer   Ideally, during the first three months of pregnancy there should be no increase in weight. During the next 12 weeks the correct weight-gain should be between 3– 5 kg (7– 11 lb). In the last 12 weeks a gain of 500 g (1 lb) per week is considered an ideal state of affairs. Try not to increase your weight by more than this amount.

It is important not to start a pregnancy if you are very much overweight. Women who reach term, or delivery date, weighing over 90 kg (200 lb) have a 30 to 40 per cent increased risk of toxaemia of pregnancy, and are three to four times more likely to have a stillbirth or lose their baby shortly after birth. They also experience slightly increased mortality risks themselves.

Weight-gain in pregnancy

Question   What makes up the normal increases in body weight during pregnancy, apart from the baby? Is it all due to fat?

Answer   No, it is not all due to fat. The placenta, or afterbirth, the increased size of the womb and the amniotic fluid in which the baby floats account for 2 kg (4½ lb). The breasts weigh an extra 750 g (1½ lb) and the mother has an extra 500 g (1 lb) of circulatory blood. If she has a 3.2 kg (7 lb) baby, this adds up to about 6.3 kg (14 lb). She should also gain about 2.25– 4 kg (5– 9 lb) of extra fat stored on the body. This may be looked upon as a milk fat storage organ. If a woman breastfeeds her baby this extra fat is used up quite quickly in the course of milk production. If the baby is bottlefed or weaned early, this extra weight tends to stick unless it is lost by following a suitable diet.

Age factor

Question   Is it more difficult to lose weight as you get older?

Answer   Yes, particularly if you have become less active. There is no doubt in the minds of many doctors, although there is no convincing scientific evidence to prove it, that fat which has become 'an old friend' is loathe to leave you. But there are other factors which operate in another direction. Older people are usually more patient and persevering than younger people. This makes their slower weight-loss on the diet of their choice easier to come to terms with. Success comes slowly but easily.

Infertility

Question   Is it true that obesity can cause infertility?

Answer   Yes, there is a relationship with infertility as far as female obesity is concerned. The very fat woman, like the very thin woman, often suffers an irregular or absent ovulation and this is reflected in irregular or absent periods. When this is the case, infertility may occur.

It is important to be sure that we are talking about natural menstruation in this context. The monthly bleeding induced by the routine of oral contraception is an entirely false type of menstruation called withdrawal bleeding. Once an oral contraceptive is stopped there is no guarantee that menstruation will establish itself rapidly, whatever your weight. In fact, there is usually a period of infertility after stopping the pill. In some instances this may be prolonged.

Menopause

Question   Can the menopause cause obesity?

Answer   There are several factors operating at the menopause, some of which are discussed in the section on glandular obesity. In addition, fluid retention (swelling of fingers, ankles and elsewhere) often makes itself felt. Broadly speaking, hormone replacement therapy does not help but diuretic tablets do.

Due to an inexplicable reason, intestinal gas distention problems often complicate the menopause, with the result that skirts and trousers seem to 'shrink' at night. Certain foods, such as beans, cauliflower, onions and potatoes, often aggravate this problem and are best excluded from the diet. A main meal in the middle of the day rather than a large dinner in the evening sometimes helps.

Finally, there is an element of true obesity at this time, perhaps resulting from a more settled middle-age, getting up later in the morning, more leisure and more than a touch of self-indulgence. In such cases, finding and following the right diet is the cure.

New developments

Question Are there any 'breakthroughs' likely in the slimming game? I've tried everything, but just can't shift my enormous bulk.

Answer Generally speaking, the greater the 'bulk', the more difficult and prolonged is the slimming regime. However, the person who cannot be helped has not yet been born, so do not despair.

There are signs of a new type of slimming pill on the horizon. It is called Acarbose and is made by the German pharmaceutical giant, Bayer. At present it is only available in Germany. It works on a completely new principle, as far as slimming is concerned. It slows down or stops completely the digestive substances which break down carbohydrates into glucose in the upper part of the gastro-intestinal tract. In other words, it inhibits the *absorption* of carbohydrate.

One of the attractions of Acarbose as a slimming aid is that virtually none of the drug (less than one per cent) is absorbed into the bloodstream. Its action, therefore, is entirely local and all that happens is that perhaps half of all eaten carbohydrate is eliminated through the bowel. It seems, therefore, a remarkably safe drug, but this does not mean that it is free from side effects. Because large quantities of undigested carbohydrate pass into the large bowel, there is a tendency for users to develop unpleasant intestinal flatulence. The discomfort of this problem varies and is related to the amount of carbohydrate eaten. Nevertheless, abdominal pain and distension, nausea and intestinal wind are sufficiently common to make taking the drug a less than happy answer to all slimming problems. Some Acarbose enthusiasts consider these side effects an aid to carbohydrate avoidance and, therefore, a change in long term eating patterns. A carbohydrate binge is more or less certain to be followed a few hours later by a sharp reminder of diet breaking. The manufacturers of Acarbose are seeking ways of cutting down the side effects, with, apparently, some success.

Acarbose is particularly effective in reducing the digestion and absorption of cane sugar, sucrose. It allows up to 60 per cent of all ingested sucrose to be eliminated from the body, unchanged by the gut. So, when the problems have been overcome, it will be particularly useful for the sweet-toothed slimmer.

In the United States, a similar type of slimming aid is being researched. This does for fat what Acarbose does for carbohydrate. Should such a drug ever reach the market and be combined with a 'symptom free' type of Acarbose, it will, in effect, put all slimmers on to a high protein/low carbohydrate diet, whatever they eat.

Overweight and health

Question How dangerous is overweight? We all have to die some day.

Answer The 'rider' to this question is nearly always posed by those who ask for advice, but who really do not want to act upon it. The fact that we will all eventually die is often given as a 'sound reason' for not giving up smoking, not limiting alcohol intake to reasonable quantities, not dieting and not taking regular exercise.

The actual risks of being overweight are now fairly well understood. There is evidence that overweight in certain age groups is very definitely associated with certain, unarguable 'health penalties', including sudden death. In other age groups, the health hazards of obesity are less dramatic.

Fig. 1 relates to two age groups—20-29 and 30-39. Average mortality is 100 and the Body Mass Index, weight divided by height squared, is explained in Chapter I. This is significant and important, for it is these age groups that are most at risk with obesity. Fig. 2 relates Body Mass Index to wider age groups and shows that the relationship of obesity to morbidity (illness) holds good too, to some extent. Fig. 3 demonstrates the sudden death factor.

A very large survey, of 12,516 men and women, has shown that obese men are at increased risk of having a first major coronary 'event' *only* if they are under the age of 50. Between 50 and 55, overweight carries no extra risk of this and over the age of 55 there is a slight and insignificant reduction in risk. Similar age groups seem to be at risk as far as blood pressure is concerned. An association between overweight and hypertension is much stronger in the 20-39 age group than in the 40-64 age group. Further studies, which involved a wide range of diseases, confirm that Body Mass Indices of 20-25 are the most healthy and least likely to be associated with disease.

Fig. 4 shows how overweight (defined as those who paid increased insurance premiums due to being overweight) is related to various mortality rates in a wide variety of illnesses.

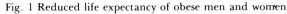

Fig. 1 Reduced life expectancy of obese men and women

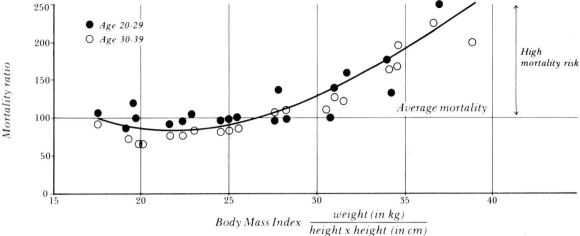

Fig. 2 Relationship of obesity in men to morbidity
(coronary thrombosis)

Fig. 3 Relationship of obesity in men to sudden death
(coronary thrombosis)

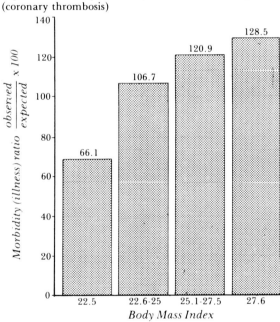

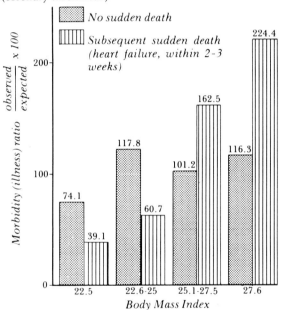

Fig. 4 Relationship of obesity to mortality rates in various illnesses

Condition	Percentage actual mortality compared with expected	
	MEN	WOMEN
Cardiovascular and renal disease	149	177
Diabetes	383	372
Cirrhosis of liver	249	177
Appendicitis	223	195
Gallstones	206	284
Pneumonia	102	129
Accidents	111	135

Cholesterol

Question Will high fat diets give me a high blood cholesterol level?

Answer The problem of cholesterol and its relationship to diet is complex and not thoroughly understood. Many simplistic fallacies have crept into the picture and many a dietary expert paints his (dietary) canvas with colours that really do not convince the medical scientist. Often genetic factors, exercise patterns and stress patterns have more effect on diseases associated with high blood cholesterol than the actual diet.

Health foods

Question Are health foods less fattening than processed foods?

Answer Yes and no. Bran is a health food and is a good aid to slimming (see the Pritikin Diet in Chapter VIII and the high fibre recipes in Chapter XIV). Honey, another health food, is very fattening. Pizzas, which are processed foods, are also fattening but other processed foods, such as frozen fish or unsweetened fruit juices, are useful items on any diet sheet.

Carbohydrates

Question Are all carbohydrates equally fattening?

Answer No. Even if reduced to a common calorific denomination (i.e. if you eat 500 calories of 'fuel', whatever the food), the complex highly fibrous carbohydrates are less fattening than the simple, or empty, ones such as sugar and syrup (see the Pritikin Diet in Chapter VIII and the high fibre recipes in Chapter XIV).

Proprietary slimming foods

Question Is a permanent diet of proprietary slimming foods a safe way to lose weight?

Answer It depends on what you mean by 'permanent'. Long periods on any artificial food cut across all the premises of good nutrition. Anybody who opts to stay on a long-term dietary project compounded around proprietary slimming foods probably needs good psychiatric as well as adequate nutritional advice.

Surgery

Question What are the possibilities of having an operation to get slim? I'm told it is very effective but risky.

Answer Surgery is usually limited to people who suffer from massive obesity, such as a weight greater than 200 per cent of their ideal weight. Such obesity affects both the quality and length of life.

On most diets, it takes a year to lose 50 kg (110 lb) and many very obese people need to lose much more than this. Unfortunately, the excessively obese are not very often able to comply with dietary stringency and, even if they do, they seem to have a built-in tendency to regain their lost weight very quickly. With such a depressing outlook, many turn their eyes hopefully towards surgery. Losing some weight 'at a stroke' or, perhaps more significantly, 'at a slice', is rarely possible, although limited amounts of fat can be removed from the abdomen. More important, perhaps, is the clever way in which surgeons can 'tidy up' the superfluous folds of skin, which continue to give nasty flabby reminders of previous obesity after weight has been lost. Most surgical methods of slimming however, are merely mechanical ways of obtaining the calorie deficit that is so necessary for weight-loss in the majority of cases.

Five techniques are currently fashionable. Dental splinting involves literally wiring the jaws together to make feeding a chore. Also, only a very restricted diet can be managed. The operation is carried out under a local anaesthetic and it is quite safe. Provided the slimmer has sound teeth, it can be done at any age. The lack of jaw movement prevents proper mastication and difficulties in mouth cleaning lead to dental decay. However, the procedure is easily reversible. Although a satisfactory weight-loss can be guaranteed in about 70 per cent of cases, the long-term success rate is poor and weight is quickly regained.

Truncal vagotomy is a relatively simple operation which divides the nerves that supply the stomach. The stomach, subsequently, functions poorly and tends to 'sag' and retain food, with the result that early satiety reduces food intake. However, for many people, the feeling is so unpleasant or even intolerable, they quickly return to their surgeons. A surgical solution to these nasty feelings is not a technical problem, but the appetite soon increases and the lost weight is inevitably regained.

Gastric partition divides the stomach to produce one area which food does not enter and a small pouch from which food travels to the small intestine for further digestion. A 30 per cent weight-loss can be expected. Afterwards, only small meals can be eaten and vomiting occurs if a heavy meal is attempted. This type of major surgery is unsuitable for people over the age of 50. Unlike by-pass operations (see below), serious, long-term side effects do not occur, but the operation carries a three per cent mortality rate.

By-pass operations join the stomach to the small bowel, so that nearly half its length is effectively by-passed. A 30 per cent weight-loss is quite likely.

Unfortunately, such operations are often followed by long-term, nutritional side effects. Diarrhoea and abdominal distension, salt balance problems, joint pains, skin rashes, brittle bones, liver damage and anal problems are fairly frequent complications. Sometimes side effects become intolerable or pose a serious threat to life, so that reversal procedures have to be carried out.

Like gastric partition, by-pass operations are unsuitable for people over 50. The mortality rate is thought to be between two and four per cent. However, before condemning such surgery as excessively risky to life, it must be noted that many of the people who undergo it are already at a high risk of dying because of their obesity.

There are various new operations currently being evaluated. These either separate digestive juices from the intestinal contents or combine this 'juice by-pass' with an operation to reduce the size of the stomach. This complicated surgery is said to produce considerable weight-loss without the more serious complications of bowel by-pass. Time alone will show how effective and safe such techniques are.

All surgical procedures, with the possible exception of the newer digestive juice by-pass operation, produce weight-loss mainly by reducing food intake. Most experts today think that there is an upper weight limit of 150 kg (331 lb). Surgery is too risky for people heavier than this.

Vitamins

Question Is it important to take vitamins when I am dieting?

Answer Yes. See Chapter I for full details.

Bowel movements

Question Will frequent bowel movements make me lose weight?

Answer At least one bogus slimming treatment was based on this premise (see Chapter XIII). In fact, a dose of saline laxatives, or purging salts such as Glauber's and Epsom salts, will be reflected in a quick flick of the scales in the direction of weight-loss. This is due to body fluid loss because such laxatives work by withdrawing fluids from the tissues as well as retaining the liquid part of bowel contents. The body is, however, quick to adjust to assaults on its natural fluid balance and fairly soon the body fluid state is back in equilibrium and the scales return to normal. Frequent bowel motions on high bulk, or fibre, diets produce a slight but probably infinitesimal contribution to slimming in terms of body heat loss.

Fasting

Question Is it dangerous to fast?

Answer The short, three-day, fast described in Chapter IV is safe enough. Prolonged fasting leads to a state of malnutrition and people gradually look like the inhabitants of a concentration camp. Clearly, this is dangerous to health.

Grapefruit diets

Question How effective are 'grapefuit' diets?

Answer There is no consistent definition of a grapefruit diet. But any diet that relies on a particularly bizarre formula seems doomed to failure on a long-term basis (see Chapter VIII, Bogus diets).

Homoeopathic treatment

Question Can homoeopathic treatment help me to lose weight?

Answer Yes, homoeopathic treatment can help in weight-loss. As mentioned in Chapter I, stress both in adults and children is very closely tied up with obesity. A homoeopathic physician takes a very full medical history from his patient and then carefully evaluates the personal stress situation. Homoeopathic medicine is highly individual and there is no special homoeopathic 'slimming pill' or diet. Each overweight person is treated primarily with what homoeopathists call that person's own 'constitutional remedy', which is based on an analysis relating to personality and symptoms.

Anorexia nervosa

Question What is anorexia nervosa? Is it caused by crazy dieting?

Answer Anorexia nervosa is basically a psychological problem in which someone, usually a teenage girl, finds herself acutely unhappy about her present predicament. In many cases, worries about sexual maturation are involved and the young adolescent takes an aversive dislike to her changed and nubile state. By food avoidance and self-induced vomiting she reduces her weight to such an extent that her periods stop and she virtually becomes a child again. Powerful factors are usually involved in anorexia nervosa and some psychiatrists believe that the best method of management is by family group-psychotherapy.

'Crazy dieting', which is something that many teenagers go in for now and again, seldom if ever leads to anorexia nervosa. This type of dieting usually makes people feel very hungry and often quite ill. They then have a good meal and feel better. Hopefully, if they are overweight they will find a suitable and sensible diet to follow.

Smoking and diets

Question I've been ordered to give up smoking because of a coronary. People tell me that, if I do, I will get fat. I believe that I'm just in the healthy range as far as my weight is concerned, but if I increase weight won't I be just as badly off as I was before?

Answer There is no doubt that there are considerable differences in weight between smokers and non-smokers. A survey of a group of middle-aged steel workers showed that life-long non-smokers are 5.9 kg (13 lb) heavier than the smokers of the same age. People almost inevitably put on weight when they give up smoking and there are several reasons for this.

Many hazards of smoking are unrelated to obesity. For example, tar from tobacco produces lung cancer and cadmium and other chemicals destroy elastic tissues, leading to chronic bronch-itis and emphysema. However, many other body changes due to smoking are associated with fat storage. Someone who smokes about 20 cigarettes a day reduces his blood's capacity to carry oxygen by about 10 per cent. Most people learn to cope, over the years, with blood circulating in their bodies at 90 per cent efficiency. This probably has a small, but constant, effect on metabolic processes, which all rely on oxygen for their efficiency. It may be, therefore, that fat build-up is adversely affected by this inefficiency, which is good news as far as obesity is concerned.

By far the most important effect of smoking on weight is related to the nicotine in tobacco. This powerful drug has a dual action on the central nervous system, the brain and nerves of the body, acting first as a stimulant and then as a depressant. However, as well as affecting the mood, nicotine also affects the stomach. Normally, appetite and feelings of hunger are associated with contractions of the stomach. It is likely that there is an appetite centre in the brain which helps to control or stimulate these contractions. They are partly habitual—you feel hungry at lunchtime and not in the middle of the night—and the burst of activity from the appetite centre at such times normally lasts for about 15 minutes. However, a small amount of nicotine (one cigarette) can abolish hunger contractions for at least 15 minutes and often longer.

This is not the only anti-eating factor built into the habit of smoking. Nicotine can reduce the volume and the acidity of the gastric juice. In a poorly functioning stomach, food is slowly digested and inadequately absorbed. Most of the effects of nicotine are quickly reversible once the drug is discontinued. The plight of the ex-smoker and his weight is, therefore, fairly predictable. First, his blood starts to function rather more efficiently. He feels hungrier and if, like many confirmed tobacco addicts, he used to smoke between courses, then his appetite will return with an unexpected zest. Moreover, the new-found efficiency of his stomach will demand more food.

On top of all these problems is another, perhaps the most difficult to cope with—a unique feeling of deprivation and loss of purpose associated with giving up smoking. We have already looked at the psychological tendencies to equate food with comfort, security, being loved and 'wanted'. The dieter has to make readjustments to cope with the anxious and depressed feeling of being deprived of these pleasures of life.

The smoker has also come to regard nicotine as an old and trusted friend to help him cope with everyday stresses and strains. To remove successfully these two comforting props at the same time, the dieting ex-smoker needs a really high motivation, such as not having another heart attack. Weight reduction and giving up smoking should not be attempted simultaneously, unless there is a very pressing, usually medical, reason. In effect, the real answer to the question is, unless overweight is really excessive, stopping smoking gives the greatest health bonus.

Sex and slimming

Question   Is it true that sex is a good way to lose weight?

Answer   You need to have a great deal of sex to lose a little weight. But there is no doubt that all exercise, together with some minor physiological factors, will ease the scales in the right direction. Perhaps it would be safer to say that a lot of extra sex may help you to lose a little extra weight.

Stretch marks

Question   Will I get stretch marks if I lose weight?

Answer   You may experience stretch marks as your weight *increases*. These look a reddish brown colour at this stage. As you shrink with effective dieting, the stretch marks first become blueish and then turn an unobtrusive silvery grey. The development of stretch marks varies considerably from person to person, both in obesity and in pregnancy.

Hormones

Question   Do hormone injections help with slimming? I've heard they get the fat off just the right places.

Answer   Spot dieting is a delusion. Injections of a hormone called human chorionic gonadotrophin (HCG) have been popular in rather way-out slimming clinics for some time. The only ones that have published successful results also maintained their clients on a 500 calorie diet for six weeks! Other exotic claims were made for HCG and it was said to increase libido and fertility, arrest hair loss, improve the voice and even help

with painful periods. Dispassionate observers suggest that the sheer act of having an injection, not what was actually injected, plus the ketosis inherent in the 500 calorie diet was what really affected the slimmers. In other words, the action is a *placebo* effect.

Cold weather

Question   Do I need to eat more food in cold weather?

Answer   Your body certainly needs to produce more heat if your environment is cold, *provided* you do not efficiently insulate yourself against the cold with extra clothes or central heating. Most people pile on more clothes and turn up the heating, so 'stoking up' with pies and puddings on a cold winter's day can be counter-productive to effective slimming.

Drinking with meals

Question   Is drinking with meals bad for my diet?

Answer   It depends what you drink. Water or low-calorie drinks are acceptable, in any quantity. Most alcoholic drinks contain empty calories and increase the appetite. Most diets with a real weight-loss in mind are alcohol-free.

Salt on food

Question   Does putting a lot of salt on my food prevent weight-loss?

Answer   In a state of good health, no. The body automatically gets rid of excess salt in the diet by excreting it into the urine. If, however, you suffer from a fluid retention condition, which is especially common in women who experience the premenstrual syndrome, then salt sometimes aggravates this. Body fluid, not fat, is retained in this way and a low salt diet or a diuretic, or water producing pill, will act as a corrective.

Diuretics

Question   Do diuretics help weight-loss?

Answer   Diuretics only help weight-loss if excess weight is produced by excess fluid retained in the body tissue.

Index

Note: Numbers in italics denote recipes.